A DAUGHTER'S PERSPECTIVE

NURSING HOME 101

BY RUTHIE ROSAUER

Copyright © 2021 by Ruth Rosauer

ISBN: 978-1-7361714-9-3

Rosauer. Ruth
Nursing Home 101: A Daughter's Perspective.

Edited by: Melissa Long

Warren publishing

Published by Warren Publishing
Charlotte, NC
www.warrenpublishing.net
Printed in the United States

*This book is dedicated to my husband, Mark,
who has been my rock-solid support throughout the
nursing home years, and the writing of this book.*

Table of Contents

Introduction 1
CHAPTER ONE Choosing a Nursing Home 7
CHAPTER TWO Bedsores and Pressure Ulcers 27
CHAPTER THREE Attention! Attention! 33
CHAPTER FOUR Swallowing Issues 51
CHAPTER FIVE Baths 63
CHAPTER SIX Visiting... 71
CHAPTER SEVEN Hearing Aids and Glasses 83
CHAPTER EIGHT Hospice...................................... 97
CHAPTER NINE Grooming 129
CHAPTER TEN Paperwork 145
CHAPTER ELEVEN More Frustrations.................... 171
CHAPTER TWELVE Staff 191
CHAPTER THIRTEEN Coming to the End 203
The Need for Reform 225
Conclusion.. 249
Acknowledgments 251
Endnotes 253

Introduction

The hospital's social worker found us in Mom's room and motioned for us to come into the hallway. "What are your plans?" she asked.

Jenny and I looked at each other with bewilderment. "Plans?"

"Plans for your mother. She is being discharged tomorrow. What do you plan to do with her?"

My sister and I were in complete shock. We were still waiting for someone to sit down with us and tell us just what her situation was. We thought someone would be giving us the complete medical picture, a possible prognosis, and a recommended roadmap for her future care. We had never had any experience with transient ischemic attacks (TIAs) or strokes. Everyone in our family to this point had died from cancer or a heart attack, so these were uncharted waters for us. This was the first we had heard that she would be discharged the next day.

"We don't have a plan," we admitted.

"Well, you need to get a plan," the social worker huffed. "You can't expect her to stay in the hospital! Can one of you take her home with you?"

With that inauspicious conversation, my sister and I were dropped headfirst into the often hostile and always bewildering world of long-term care facilities. My mother was in a nursing home in New Jersey from 2006 until she died in January 2010. I was living in Wisconsin during this period, and my sister lived in northern New York State.

My mother and I had never been close. In fact, we had gone for long periods of time without speaking to each other. We come from a long line of people who cut family members out of their lives. We were good at it and comfortable with it. If you had told me prior to my mother's stroke that I would jump in my car and drive one thousand miles to help take care of her, I would have said you were mistaken.

But when I got the call that she was in the hospital, there was no hesitation on my part. The pull to her was unmistakable, as though I were a fish who thought she had been swimming freely, blissfully unaware of the hook imbedded in her mouth. And when the yank came on that hook in the form of that phone call, I had no other thoughts—I just followed. With my mom's stroke, I learned I had been securely bound to her all along.

I keep a journal, so I have many contemporaneous entries from that period. The order of these chapters reflects, roughly, the order in which we encountered particular issues with our mother's tenure in the nursing home.

Please note that the stroke my mother suffered three months after her TIA left her with aphasia—a great difficulty in speaking. She was unable to form a complete sentence until a full year, almost to the day, after her stroke. Even then, her language was never normal again. There would be long pauses, pieces of words, garbled words, gestures, and more, and I would guess to ascertain her intention. She would let me know when I had guessed correctly. I thought readers would be frustrated if I painstakingly recreated her vocal efforts for the entire length of this book. She regained neither her full vocabulary, nor the flow of her words, even if it may appear that way from the way I've written some of the dialogue in this book. Her loss of verbal fluency exacerbated many of her difficulties in dealing with the health-care staff.

I had hoped nursing homes would have improved their quality of service since my mother's death in 2010 and therefore, render my story irrelevant today, make it of interest only to myself and my sister. I am a Senior Tar Heel Legislator for my county in North Carolina. One of our issues for lobbying the state legislature in 2019 was staffing of nursing homes. When I spoke with my acquaintances about the Senior Tar Heel's issues, I found several people who wanted to share their experiences about loved ones in nursing homes, some of those being as recent as 2019. After hearing their stories, I decided there is, indeed, still a need for this book.

All names of health-care providers, including facilities, have been changed in this book, as have all names of those interviewed about their experiences with nursing homes.

I know the preferred term is "skilled nursing facility" instead of "nursing home." I find the former term confuses people as it generally conjures images of patients in a burn recovery unit or in an intensive care unit with tubes, wires, and beeping monitors, so I tend to use "nursing home." I use "long-term care" as an umbrella term for "nursing homes," "skilled-nursing units," and "assisted-living facilities."

* * *

The world of long-term care facilities for seniors is a relatively new one. Atul Gawande outlined the history of care for the elderly in the United States in his book, *Being Mortal: Medicine and What Matters in the End*.[1] Nursing homes in the United States originated in the 1950s when hospitals requested government help in removing elderly and frail patients with nowhere else to go from hospital beds. By 1970, thanks to government funding, there were about thirteen thousand nursing homes. Health and safety issues were endemic from the beginning.

Nursing homes are like lawyers in that most people avoid them if possible. People often dislike visiting residents in the facilities, and many people would go for three root canals rather than live in one. Yet, in 2019, there were about 1.4 million people living in 15,500 nursing homes in the United States. The Centers for Disease Control and Prevention estimates there will be approximately three million residents in nursing homes by 2030.[2]

When you are thrown into the world of long-term care, you have a lot on your plate—probably a car to sell, personal belongings to dispose of, a house to sell, medical questions to research, and an ocean of emotional issues. Hopefully, this book will educate you about skilled care facilities and alert you to potential issues you may be able to forestall or ameliorate with adequate information and planning.

Each chapter opens with my experience with my mom, then broadens with the experiences of others on the same topic. Each continues with a section I call "For the Record," with statistics and medical and regulatory information pertinent to the subject. When possible, I end a chapter with tips for others.

My fondest hope is that this book may spark significant systemic changes to the nursing home industry. As a former marketing director at a nursing-home told me, "It is certainly a broken system. It desperately needs to be fixed." Over one million Americans are depending on us to do so. One of those residents could be your mom or dad—or even you yourself!

CHAPTER 1
Choosing a Nursing Home

I received a call one afternoon telling me my mother had suffered a transient ischemic attack (TIA) and was in the hospital. It took me twenty-one hours to drive from my house in Wisconsin to the hospital in New Jersey. Jenny, my sister, who was living only seven hours away, got there first. This was the first time my mother had been a patient in a hospital since she had given birth to Jenny fifty years earlier. When I arrived at her room, she was obviously in misery. She was mentally confused and unable to say the day of the week or her home address. She hadn't called Jenny by name and didn't seem to recognize me either. She didn't understand why she was in the hospital. One thing she did communicate frequently was her wish to go home.

The staff described her TIA as a small stroke. If this was a small stroke, I couldn't imagine what a big one would be like. A small stroke looked pretty major to me.

The second day, I arrived at the hospital early enough to catch the night-shift nurse as she was leaving. "Your mother was pretty bad last night," she told me. "I don't know how she did it, but she slipped out of bed and took her clothes off. We found her crawling down the hallway naked. We put her back in bed with wrist restraints so she wouldn't get out again."

I entered her room and saw Mom was held fast to her bed with white, plastic rings encircling her tiny wrists. When she woke up, her eyes were shooting venom. "I want out of this place," she seethed.

"Mom," I said soothingly, "we're just trying to figure out what is going on with you. You'll be out soon."

Three days later, the hospital's social worker found us in Mom's room and gave us the shocking news that we needed a placement for our mother within twenty-four hours. After we explained that neither of us lived within five hundred miles of our mother, the social worker probed for other possibilities.

"Don't you have any other family who could take her?" she demanded.

My sister and I exchanged glances before I spoke. "All she has left is one sister, and she is eighty-nine years old."

"Then you'd better find a rehabilitation center for her."

Stunned, I asked, "Can you recommend one?"

"I already contacted St. Joseph and they say they won't take her. They are very selective about who they take. You could try Pineville or Meadow Crest. They would have to send someone out to evaluate her first, so you need to move fast."

We had cell phones, but they weren't working inside the hospital. Jenny and I scrambled for change for the payphone and contacted Pineville. They said their social worker was at the hospital already and could come by and evaluate Mom in an hour. My mind was still reeling with the thought that my mom had flunked one rehabilitation center. How could this be? Was it her age? Were they too crowded already? Had her SAT scores not been high enough? Did they think she wasn't otherwise physically fit enough? I had never had any dealings with a rehabilitation center, and therefore, no notion they would even have a criteria for accepting a patient. If I had given it any thought before then, I would have assumed a rehabilitation center was like a hospital emergency room—if they had space, they had to take you! Boy, did I have a lot to learn!

It turned out that Pineville had an opening and thought Mom was an appropriate patient for them. The Pineville social worker was very nice to my mom. After she left, Mom said, "That lady must have a really big house. She wants me to come live with her for a while. She says there are other patients there too." Mom thought she was going to a private home and not a rehabilitation center, but that was okay with us. We had anticipated a knock-down, drag-out fight when she found out she wasn't going back to her apartment.

Mom improved enough in the rehab center that she did eventually return to her apartment. We arranged for a home health aide to come three times a week, a private-pay companion to visit her every day, and delivery of lunch by Meals on Wheels.

What we didn't know, and what her doctors had failed to tell us, was the likelihood that Mom would have another stroke within ninety days. With subsequent research, I learned that 12–20 percent of all those experiencing a TIA will have a stroke or heart failure, within ninety days. Age is a risk factor in this forecast, so at eighty-eight years old, my mother would have had a 20 percent chance to have a larger stroke within ninety days.[3] No one ever even hinted that we should take this factor into consideration.

As it turned out, she was home for only three months.

JOURNAL ENTRY 1-2

I didn't like to call my mom too early because she didn't get up until nine o'clock or so, and then it took her quite a while to dress. Juanita, her home health aide, poured her cereal into a bowl each night before she left and put a little milk in a small, plastic bottle in the refrigerator. This way, Mom didn't have to wrestle with a big, heavy container of milk.

I first called her around ten o'clock in the morning. There was no answer. She had two cordless phones and always kept one in the basket on her walker. Maybe she was taking a shower. Maybe she forgot to recharge both phones. I kept calling and leaving messages on her answering machine.

Jenny called me at noon. She, too, had been unsuccessful in reaching Mom. We had gotten Mom a button-activated alert device to wear on a cord around her neck. If she pressed the emergency call button, it was supposed to send an ambulance. Although they told her it was waterproof, she insisted on taking it off when she took a shower. What if she had fallen in the shower?

We decided to call her neighbor, Joe, to ask him to check on Mom. Thankfully, Joe was home and cheerfully agreed to go check on her. I waited twenty minutes and called him back. No answer. I called my mom's apartment again. Joe answered my mom's phone. "She's just lying there on the couch. She's not moving!" He sounded panicked.

"Joe, did you call 911?"

"No. She didn't answer the door. I went to her window and looked in. I saw her on the couch. I broke in through the window. She's not answering me!" Joe was frantic.

"Joe," I enunciated as clearly as I could, "I'm going to hang up now, and I want you to dial 911, okay?"

"Yeah," he said. "I told her to leave her door unlocked so I could check on her. Why didn't she leave her door unlocked?"

"Please, Joe, call 911, okay?"

"Yeah," he said, and I hung up so he could.

I called my sister and told her what happened. "Did you tell Joe that Mom's medical information is in the big, brown envelope on the coffee table and marked 'Hazel's medical information' in big letters? Did you tell him to put it on the stretcher with her?"

"No!" I felt terrible. How could I have forgotten that?

"Did you tell him to take her to St. Thomas hospital and not the city hospital?"

"Oh God, I forgot!" I was an idiot! What else had I forgotten? "Jenny, please, call Mom's apartment right now. Maybe the ambulance is still there. I'll call Joe's phone in case he went back home."

Jenny caught Joe just as the paramedics were wheeling Mom out. Despite Jenny's request, they failed to take the envelope. Mom went to the hospital without a friend, relative, or any identification.

"Jenny, it just occurred to me that she might be dead. Do you think she might be dead?"

Jenny chose not to speculate about this over the phone.

A few hours later Jenny called the hospital. "We can't give patient information over the phone."

"But I'm her daughter, and I have her power of attorney!" Jenny wailed.

"We can't give out patient information on the phone. To anyone."

Jenny and I called everyone we knew in our hometown to see if someone would go check on her in person. We were distraught to think of her lying there on a gurney in that big hospital emergency room without anyone to tell her where she was or to get her a blanket if she was cold. We knew firsthand what that hospital was like from Mom's ministroke back in April. It was not the warm and fuzzy place that hospitals are cracked up to be.

Mom still lived in the town where Jenny and I had been born. But I hadn't lived there since 1975, and Jenny hadn't lived there for the previous ten years. Still, we knew a few names and phone numbers. Jenny's in-laws were our first choice, but there was no answer there. No answer at Juanita's either. We struck out a few more times until my sister reached someone who went to my mom's church—Rick.

"Sure," he said, "I'll go right over."

Rick called my sister back on his cellphone later. "Your mom is still in the emergency room. They say she's had another stroke. They think she's going to live, but they missed the three-hour window for giving her that medication for strokes. It looks like her left side is paralyzed. I'm going to stay with her until they decide what is going on."

My sister thanked Rick profusely. Then she thought to ask, "How did you get into the emergency room to see her?"

"Easy. I just told them I was her son. Nobody asked me for any ID."

Eventually, after a phone call the next day from Mom's doctor, we found out that she had suffered a stroke, a major one this time. It affected the left side of her body and the muscles in her throat. It was too soon to tell if she would be able to talk again. They admitted her to the hospital. Jenny arrived the next day.

JOURNAL ENTRY 1-3

Jenny called to give me another update on Mom. "The stroke has affected the muscles in her throat. She can't swallow anything. Not even water. She chokes trying to drink water. Can you believe it? They gave her something called a swallow test. She can't eat or drink anything. They have her on an IV right now, but they say they are going to put a stomach tube in her for feeding."

"Okay," I said. "I'll be there Saturday. I bought my plane ticket. I'll get online and do some research on feeding tubes and stuff."

Putting in a feeding tube. The procedure sounded so routine the way Jenny said it that it didn't even set off any alarm bells in my head. But they started to clang loudly as I read on the internet that the insertion of a feeding tube in the stomach is a serious decision. It should only be made after a careful and complete discussion with the family, patient, and doctor. I ran to my desk and pulled out my copy of my mother's advance medical directive—in some states, these are called "living wills." Sure enough, she had checked the box indicating she didn't want to be kept alive by artificial means. The stomach feeding tube was specifically mentioned as something she did not want. And the doctor hadn't even talked to me or Jenny about it; he had only left a message on Jenny's answering machine.

I called her back. "Jenny, I know I promised you I would never second-guess any decision you would make about Mom. I know you might have to make split-second decisions and that you'll do the best you can. But

I have to tell you, this stomach tube is a *huge* decision. The internet says it has moral implications. This would definitely be keeping her alive by artificial means. Did the doctor talk to you *at all* about this?"

Jenny confirmed that her only information about it was a voicemail message from the doctor saying the procedure was planned for the next day. We talked about it at length and agreed that, as far as we knew, it was too early to know what kind of recovery Mom may be able to make. Still, if she wasn't able to eat, she would surely die in a few days. We decided to let them put in the stomach tube to buy her a little more time so the professionals could assess her chances of recovery. We didn't want to sentence her to a premature death if she was capable of recovering a decent quality of life. We were willing, provided the feeding tube was reversible. Jenny said there was a social worker assigned to Mom's case, and she would try to reach her and ask about it. The social worker said the stomach tube was very routine, posed little risk, and was most certainly reversible. Jenny and I agreed to let them do the surgery the next day.

JOURNAL ENTRY 1-4

"Why didn't you let me go?" my mother asked me with obvious effort. Her pronunciation was muddy, the question garbled and labored. I wasn't sure I'd heard her correctly. This was her first sentence to me since her stroke, and I would have been thrilled with her having put together an entire sentence if it hadn't been for the content. I pretended not to know what she meant. "Go? Do you mean 'go' as in 'go to the bathroom?'"

She shook her head left and right. She was irritated because I didn't understand her, and she didn't have the energy to try again. But this was too important to let go. I needed to know what she wanted. We had never had a conversation about her death.

"Do you mean 'go' as in 'die?'" I felt bold using this word with my mother. "Die" felt as forbidden to me as a four-letter word. She had always preferred euphemisms for death, bodily functions, and sex. Actually, she preferred not to discuss these topics at all. The stroke, however, stripped her of the ability to convey meaning by nuance, euphemism, or inference.

"Yeth," she lisped back.

I called my sister into the room to listen. I wanted her to hear this too. Mom proceeded to tell us, in her tiny, halting, rasping voice, that she had been in the process of dying on Labor Day when she was interrupted. But "interrupted" is too difficult a word for Mom. Instead, she said, "Knock, knock, knock," and then went quiet.

She had our full attention. We desperately wanted to hear the story of her stroke from her perspective. We

prodded her: "What was going 'knock, knock, knock?'"
Her eyes remained closed. We asked her again.

"They came and got me. Knock, knock, knock." She
was clearly exhausted from this effort to communicate.

"Mom, do you mean, on the day you had your
stroke, they were knocking on your door?"

"Yeth." She nodded. After a long pause, she
asked, "Wah?"

We explained again that she couldn't have water, that
the stroke had robbed her of her ability to swallow. We
told her if she drank water, it would go down into her
lungs and she would get pneumonia. This was something
we'd already explained several times. I tried to use the
same words each time, hoping the repetition would
eventually form a memory, which would then become
knowledge in her.

"The day the men came with the ambulance and
took you to the hospital, do you remember what you
were doing?"

Her eyes stayed closed. "I was passing over."

I doubt I was able to keep the excitement out of my
voice. "Mom, did you think you were going to heaven?
Did you see bright lights? Did you see Grandmom?"

"Peath."

"Mom, did you think you were dying?"

"Yeth." I waited for more. I wanted to hear all about
it, but I was afraid her exhaustion and brain damage
would prevent her from telling me. Then, very quietly,
she offered garbled words that I untangled: "Why didn't
you let me go?"

"You wanted to die?"

"Yeth."

"Mom, what were you thinking? Were you afraid?"

"No thinking." Long pause. "No thinking. Nice." She paused again, and I considered my next question, but she interrupted my train of thought. "Knock, knock, knock."

My sister and I looked at each other with sadness. It had been our phone call to Joe that had brought on the "knock, knock, knock" she found so offensive. If we hadn't called Joe, she would have been dead by the time Juanita got there to fix her supper that evening.

"Mommy, we are so sorry. We thought maybe you had fallen and were in pain. We didn't know you were dying. We called your neighbor Joe. It was Joe who knocked on your door. When you didn't answer, he went outside and broke in through your window. You were unconscious, so he called 911."

All I could do was apologize. "I'm so sorry, Mommy, that we did that."

She was already asleep, and she slept until we left that evening.

Back in the car, Jenny and I looked at each other. "Great," I said. "We saved our mother's life, and now she's mad at us for *that!*" I had felt guilty when I began to say it, but once the words were spoken, they sounded so funny, Jenny and I laughed over them for a long time. It was the first time we'd laughed since Mom had her big stroke.

JOURNAL ENTRY 1-5

Today, they transferred my mother from the hospital back to Pineville. Since her stroke on Labor Day, she'd been unable to swallow, even her own saliva. She'd not been able to sit up on her own either. The physical therapists had made one visit to her hospital room, and they got her on her feet once for about thirty seconds.

When Mom's transport arrived to take her to the nursing home, it consisted of an old man pushing a wheelchair. He looked in need of the wheelchair himself. My mother had not yet even sat in a wheelchair. My sister and I threw a fit and said there was no way we would let them bundle our mother into a wheelchair for her journey through the hospital, plunk her—still in her wheelchair—into a van, and drive her like Granny Clampett to the nursing home. The hospital floor nurse finally arrived and agreed with us. He called those in charge of transport, and an hour later two men showed up with a gurney. Mom was then transported by an ambulance-type vehicle to the nursing home.

My sister and I were aghast when we thought about what would have happened had we not been there. My mother could barely speak. You had to listen closely and guess to ascertain her meaning. She was unable to defend herself against this type of bureaucratic mix-up. Later, after we arrived at Pineville, the social worker telephoned and apologized for the wheelchair initially sent for Mom. "I don't know how it happened," she said. "I knew your mother couldn't ride in a wheelchair, and yet somehow, I ordered it anyway. I honestly don't know why. I don't know what I was thinking."

Was this supposed to be an apology? I knew what she was worried about—that we would report her to some authority and get her in trouble for this mistake. From what I'd already seen of the hospital and nursing home, I knew a mix-up in transportation was only a blip on the map of problems we'd face before my mother's death.

I was (and still am) grateful my sister and I were there and caught the error, so it was only a close call, and there was no harm done. We knew already we needed to pick our battles carefully, or we'd exhaust ourselves and earn a reputation as "difficult." I didn't plan to go to battle over this one, so I told the social worker not to worry about it.

REPORTS FROM OTHERS

"The first thing you need to know is not to base your choice of a nursing home on how nice the place looks. The first place I chose had a big front porch with rockers, nice carpet in the entryway, a wreath on the front door—that kind of thing," said Samantha, whose husband had lived with dementia. She went on to chronicle some of the problems she encountered there: his watch was stolen his first day, the only activity offered was bingo, and a leak in the roof caused a large puddle of water in his room, which no one bothered to mop up.

To deal with the lack of activities, she sought out the activity director to ask about planning some activities other than bingo. Samantha suggested they could reach out to community groups for entertainment, but she was told it took too much work to organize those things. She also felt annoyed with staff members who promised they would get back to her after she spoke to them, but they never did. Samantha always had to initiate follow-up contacts.

After her bad experience in choosing the first facility, Samantha turned to a geriatric manager to recommend her husband's next placement, which at first, she thought to be a definite improvement. However, as her husband's dementia progressed, she noted a decline in his quality of care. She said, "Nursing homes today are just warehouses of old people. If he hadn't died when he did, I don't know what I would have done because I didn't know of another nursing home for him."

Jean Miller ran into the same time-crunch problem my sister and I had encountered in choosing a facility. Her mother had fallen, hit her head, and gone to the hospital. The hospital gave Jean only one day's notice before her mother's discharge and recommended two skilled nursing facilities. Jean chose one for her mother, but then she was very frustrated because they kept losing her mother's paperwork—Jean replaced the paperwork five times in two months. To find a different placement for her mother, she turned to a geriatric nurse consultant who was recommended by Jean's own primary care physician. The geriatric nurse consultant offered more than just recommendations. The consultant subsequently visited Jean's mother in the nursing home a few times to see how she was getting along.

Claire Johnson, who placed her mother first in an assisted living facility and later in a nursing home, advised, "Take your time in finding one. If you have a loved one who will need long-term care, I suggest you already have a facility in your mind so you know where you want to go. Get to know the staff, especially the hands-on care people. Go at varied times during the day."

Making surprise visits to a care facility before making a choice for your loved one was also suggested by Sue, a former nursing-home marketing director. "If time permits, you should just walk into a nursing home without an appointment. Ask for the marketing director and request a tour. Check for reviews online and look for a Facebook page, a website, or blog written by family members or former patients. You could even reach out to some of the medical home care facilities for an opinion because they very likely have worked with those facilities."

Linda recently moved her parents from Texas to South Carolina. Her parents had never been to South Carolina before, so they were unfamiliar with facility options. In preparation for the move, Linda and her husband visited several long-term care facilities. They made it a point to eat in the dining room of each facility they considered. Then Linda and her husband settled on four possibilities. When her parents arrived, she helped them visit the four facilities and choose where they wanted to live. She said the most important things to her parents were food, activities, and transportation. Her parents had initially resisted the move and wanted to stay in their house back in Texas. But a month after they were moved into assisted living, her dad said, "We should have done this two years ago."

FOR THE RECORD

Professionals who can help you choose a nursing home go by many titles: geriatric care manager, geriatric case manager, aging life care professional, and more. These professionals have been educated first in another profession such as social work, occupational therapy, physical therapy, nursing, gerontology, or counseling. Typically, they charge by the hour. Medicare will not pay for these services, nor will most insurance plans.

The Alzheimer's Association has a piece on their website that lists questions to ask when choosing a geriatric care manager. The National Institute on Aging provides a toll-free number for an eldercare locator (800-677-1116). The Aging Life Care Association offers training for those who want to be an aging life care professional. They also post on their website a code of ethics and standards of practice. Their website also features an easy locator; just enter your zip code and the site presents names and contact info for an aging life care professional near you.

TIPS

- Don't be fooled by a nice exterior and entry area of a nursing home.
- Be prepared. If you have an elderly loved one, don't wait until the last minute to evaluate your options. A hospital is likely to give you only twenty-four to forty-eight hours to find a facility before discharging a patient. Take the time to visit facilities ahead of need for placement so you are familiar with the options in your area.
- Pay attention to inspection reports. The Centers for Medicare & Medicaid Services (CMS) contracts with states to do on-site inspections. These are required every nine to fifteen months under federal law. Three years' worth of these inspections must be available in the nursing home. You can also access them online at https://www.medicare.gov.
- Use a professional geriatric manager—if you can afford it—to help find the right facility.
- Make a surprise visit to the facility before you place a loved one there.
- Stop and listen when you visit a nursing home before placement. Is it noisy and chaotic? Noise is one of the seven red flags to watch for in choosing a nursing home because it can enhance agitation among residents.[4]
- Check the outer surroundings of a nursing home. Although residents tend to spend most of their time inside, it is good to have a secure, accessible,

outdoor space that permits residents to enjoy the air, sky, and hopefully, a bit of nature in safety.

- Do not assume that because your loved one received good care in a short-term rehabilitation section they will receive similar care and amenities in the long-term section of the same facility.

- Be honest about your loved one's issues during the intake assessment. It may be tempting to downplay problems, but it is better to be forthcoming. A nursing home's inability to care for the needs of a resident is one of the few reasons permitted to a nursing home for evicting a resident. Hopefully, you can avoid an unpleasant and stressful eviction by securing an appropriate placement at the start.

- Look for online reviews. See https://www. medicare.gov. for government surveys.

CHAPTER 2
Bedsores and Pressure Ulcers

After Mom's admission, the nursing home measured Mom's bedsore during the morning shift. It was huge, gaping, purple, and raw, with a nasty bull's-eye of pus. I suspected this caused the pain "in her buttocks" my mother had complained about even before her stroke. The visiting nurse had looked at it when Mom still lived in her apartment and claimed to have seen nothing, so we thought it was all in her head. Once she'd been able to speak at all after the stroke, she'd say single words: "thirsty," "hungry," and "pain." When we asked her where the pain was, she always gestured to her lower back and buttocks. Jenny and I had asked the hospital staff to check her for injuries in those areas in case she had fallen when she was having her stroke. They claimed they could see nothing there. The nursing-home staff later told us, emphatically, that bedsores hurt a lot and could well have been the pain she'd been complaining about.

What they didn't tell us is that a bedsore can be fatal. About sixty thousand people die of bedsore complications annually.[5]

REPORTS FROM OTHERS

Betty hadn't been a certified nursing assistant (CNA) in over ten years but her mother-in-law had been in and out of facilities as recently as 2009, so she was eager to talk about the long-term care situation. She shared, "At school, we learned that people have to be gotten up and have to be turned every two hours. But the reality when you are working in a facility is that they don't do those things. It's very disheartening to have learned these things in school as best practices, and when you get on the job, you aren't given the time to implement them. There is no time to turn people."

Karen Kerrigan's story about her mother bears repeating as a cautionary tale. I believe Karen was only able to pick up on this nursing home's incompetence because she is a registered nurse (RN).

Karen related, "My mom was ninety when she died. She had been in a nursing home for about two years before she died. I visited her at least once, and usually twice, every week she was in the nursing home. Up until about two weeks before she died, she was still able to get into the car and go on outings with me. The nursing home called one day and said that my mom had cut her leg on the wheelchair that day. When they called me, I told them, 'Listen, based on her history of poor circulation—she'd had a previous problem with a pressure sore on her foot that almost resulted in her leg being amputated—you need to jump on this and be aggressive with wound care.'

"I visited her two days later. When I saw her leg with the pus spewing out of it, I raised the alarm. It took me three calls to the doctor's office—the nursing home's doctor—before I got to speak to the nurse practitioner who agreed to meet me at the nursing home at a certain time. What was very disturbing was the nurse practitioner told me she had been to the nursing home the day before and had seen my mother and *no one* had told the nurse practitioner there was a wound on my mother's leg. All the nurse practitioner had done on her previous visit was listen to my mom's heart and press on her stomach. We unwrapped that bandage on my mom's leg, and the color drained out of the nurse's face when she saw that wound. The nurse practitioner ordered wound care.

"The plan was to send her to the hospital's official wound care center for treatment every few days for debridement and soaks and whatever else they could possibly do. That was three days before my mom died. She only got to have one of those wound care treatments. When she died, I knew right away she had died of sepsis. I had been to see her, and she wasn't herself. It was the first time ever that she didn't want to go on an outing, so I knew she wasn't herself. I offered to take her out for lunch, and she said she didn't feel like it.

"Her death certificate said cause of death was 'senile dementia.' She was a little drifty, but I had a good conversation with her on my last visit, and she was with-it enough to make jokes and to be happy for a family member who had recently been elected to office. Just the week before she died, she had been with-it enough to get out to the car, go out for lunch, and go shopping. When you start to get low-grade sepsis, you just don't feel good. It is like when you are getting the flu. I think that was where she was on my last visit to her three days before she died. Total time span from when they told me she cut herself to death was two weeks."

Karen's regret was palpable as she concluded her story. "We decided not to bring a law suit. I should have demanded an autopsy. But what would that have done for her? I was exhausted. I had been visiting my mom twice a week while raising five kids and working part-time. I was so drained, I couldn't put up a fight for her. Now? Now I would have the energy to fight for her."

FOR THE RECORD

Bedsores are also called "pressure ulcers," "pressure sores," and "decubitus ulcers." The preferred term is "pressure ulcer" because pressure is the primary cause of these wounds, and beds are not always the origin of the pressure.[6] Wherever it occurs, the constant pressure on a part of the body lessens blood flow to an area. They can also be caused by the friction of clothing or bedding on fragile skin. Several conditions put a person at increased risk of pressure ulcers: cancer, stroke, multiple sclerosis, Parkinson's disease, Alzheimer's disease, diabetes, malnutrition, smoking, hip fractures, and others.[7]

It is estimated that 10 percent of nursing-home patients suffer from pressure ulcers. That works out to about one hundred fifty thousand patients in the United Statess with a pressure sore annually.[8]

Federal rules stipulate that "a resident who is admitted without pressure sores does not develop them unless it is unavoidable, and a resident with pressure sores receives the necessary treatment to promote healing, prevent infections, and new sores."[9]

TIPS

- Examine the body of your loved one yourself. If you are squeamish, try to find another family member or close friend to check the skin. Common locations of bedsores are: just above the tailbone, heels, sides of the hips, places where the back vertebrae protrude, wherever the head is in contact with the bed or pillow, and anywhere the weight is placed while sitting.[10]
- Check for warning signs of pressure ulcers: unusual changes in skin color or texture, swelling, pus, or tender areas.[11]
- Feel the temperature of the skin in areas where you suspect a pressure ulcer could be forming. Excess warmth could be a sign of inflammation. Insufficient blood flow could indicate reduced blood flow. Either one is not a good sign and should be reported.[12]
- Prevent bed sores by making sure the body does not remain in one position for more than two hours. If you spend a lot of time in a wheelchair, try to shift your weight every fifteen minutes and completely change positions every hour.
- Problem-solve with cushions and padding to change the part of the body in contact with the chair or bed.
- Use moisturizing skin lotions to help keep skin more resilient.

CHAPTER 3
Attention! Attention!

JOURNAL ENTRY 3-1

Mom's nursing-home roommate, Sophie, was in a rage when we got to Mom's room this afternoon. She said our mom had left the premises, and everyone was upset and searching for her. Our frail mother was lying in her bed with the side rails up, hooked up to her feeding tube.

"Mommy," I scolded, "where did you go today?"

My mother was visibly agitated by my accusatory tone. I was able to piece together from her words and sounds, "I didn't go anywhere without a guard."

I was getting better at teasing out information from my mother, so I probed, "Did you go someplace *with* a guard?"

"I only went to get my hair washed."

My heart broke a little to learn she perceived the staff here as her "guards," but I was also relieved she'd not turned into one of the patients who were labeled as "flight risks." I explained to Sophie, "She only went to get her hair washed."

Sophie, red-faced with anger, was straining against the lap buddy on her wheelchair. "She has to tell somebody when she goes away! She can't just go off on her own! We were worried sick about her!" Much to my amazement, Sophie continued to rant about my mother's disappearance and finally shouted, "Next time she does this, I'm going to slap her silly when I find her!" That's when Jenny and I reported Sophie's behavior to the nurses' station. We were perplexed because, until then, Sophie had been so sweet to my mom.

The aide was very concerned and immediately took Sophie to a different room. We renewed our efforts to teach my mom how to use her call button even though I had my doubts it would successfully bring her help. First, she would have to *think* to use her call button. Then, she would have to be able to find it. There was a good chance the button would be on the floor and not even on the bed. Even if it were on the bed, there would be only about a fifty-fifty chance for it to be within her reach. The aides had a habit of clipping her call button to the sheet on the head of my mom's bed, where she couldn't find or reach it. Was there any clinical reason for this location, or was it just sheer thoughtlessness?

Even if she could have thought to use her button, found and reached it, and gathered the strength to push it, Mom's final hurdle would have been waiting for someone to show up.

JOURNAL ENTRY 3-2

I felt like I was bashing my head into an iceberg today. The cold indifference of the staff was the iceberg's tip; inefficiencies and thoughtlessness comprised its base. As I sat with Mom, I felt numb.

My mother wanted to go to bed, so when a nurse's aide came into the room, I asked her to put my mother to bed. The aide's English was not easily understandable, but I finally figured out what she was saying; she was not allowed to disconnect the stomach tube from its line to the feeding pump, so she couldn't put Mom into bed. Only a nurse could do this. Realization dawned on me that the pump was off, but while it was still connected, my mom couldn't be released from her geriatric chair.

I walked down to the nurses' station and saw three staff people sitting there. Perhaps one of them would help my mother into bed, perhaps not. First, I had to figure out the correct person to ask. One of the brambles that had to be negotiated at the nursing home was figuring out who was supposed to do what.

Nurses there would not do anything that required heavy lifting or getting their hands dirty. Aides were not allowed to disconnect feeding tubes, hand out medicine of any sort, or give you any information about a patient. The lack of specific uniforms exacerbated my identification problem—both nurses and aides wore colorful scrubs, and their tops were decorated with dancing mice, balloons, or whatever struck their fancy. Oh yes, they wore name tags but—and this was a big *but*—the majority of the staff pinned their name tags so the names faced their own bodies, not outward so anyone could read them.

I was old enough to remember when nurses wore white outfits and starched, white caps. I wished they still wore something recognizable so I could have easily distinguished their roles. I also wished the name tags were readable.

Even if I could have distinguished an aide from a nurse, I still needed to figure out who my mother's specific aide or nurse was. It was not enough to remember that Miranda took care of my mom last night—the staff assignments changed often. It was also not enough to notice who came to help my mom's roommate because they often assigned different nurses and aides to each of the two patients who shared one room.

Even if I could have figured out the correct staff position and staff person's name, I still had to find the person and ask for her help as nicely as I knew how, only to have her say, "I'll be there soon." Then we would wait, often for more than an hour.

I found this whole procedure of asking for help to be extremely annoying and *difficult*. If I couldn't properly figure out who to ask for help, then how could my little mother, with her stroke-damaged brain and barely functioning mouth and throat?

Alternatively, we could have pushed the call button in my mother's room. When we did that, we listened to the constant, droning beep of the call button while we waited for at least half an hour, or sometimes, over an hour.

If my mother were in pain, I told myself, *I would charge down to the nurses' station and like Shirley MacLaine in that movie where her daughter is dying, demand action.*

As it was, my mother was in discomfort, but she was not in excruciating pain. She had often been left sitting up for nine hours when doctor's orders were for her to sit up for only three hours at a time. She was exhausted and uncomfortable. Her diaper needed to be changed. But she was not in pain, and she was not in danger of dying at that moment. It was a delicate balancing act; I didn't want to annoy the staff so much that they became even more inefficient in their dealings with my mother, and yet I wanted them to take care of her in a timely manner.

In a nursing home, I could see patients didn't get very much of what they wanted.

JOURNAL ENTRY 3-3

I brought brightly colored modeling clay and some little molds today to see if my mom would enjoy playing with them. I had noticed that since the stroke, she showed interest in touching things, especially clothes, as if she enjoyed feeling the different textures. Pressing the clay into molds would leave the impression of an animal, such as a monkey or tiger or dog.

At about one thirty, my mother said she had to go to the bathroom. I could not get her out of the wheelchair by myself, and my sister wasn't there. I went to the nurses' station to let them know my mom would like assistance in getting to the bathroom. I was polite and low-key about it. I tried not to sound demanding. I did everything but lie down on the floor in order to exhibit lack of aggression. They said they would be right down.

I went back to my mom's room and got out the clay. I hoped it would distract her during the wait for an aide. I took a cylinder of bright red clay and held it tightly in my hand for a while to warm it up and make it more pliable for my mom. I then passed the clay to her. Then I chose a tube of purple clay and worked with it myself. My mother's pinky fingers on both hands were pulled down to the palm. The pinky finger exerted tension over the ring finger, so it wasn't very useable either. I wasn't sure what my mother could actually accomplish with the clay, but my only objective had been to give her a chance to feel it in her hands. At that moment, I also hoped it would provide a diversion while we waited for the aide.

I fashioned the purple clay into a fairly flat oval shape, then pressed it into the mold of a monkey. I showed it to my mom. She thought it was pretty cool and rubbed the red clay between her two hands to make a long worm out of it. I checked the clock; fifteen minutes had passed, not long enough to go back to the nurses' station and bug someone. I pulled the bright yellow clay out of the package and worked it between my hands. Then I took the red from my mom and gave her the yellow. I compressed the red into an oval shape and molded it into a dog. I placed it next to the monkey on a paper plate. My mother looked over at the clock.

"Those nurses never come," she whined. In my opinion, she was entitled to whine. "I wait hours for those nurses to come." I knew she wasn't exaggerating. "They come quicker when you are here," she added.

I walked back to the nurses' station. "Gosh, I was wondering about my mom?" I said softly. "Could somebody come and help her out?"

"Oh dear, didn't anyone come yet? I'll page Miranda right now and tell her to go to your mom's room."

Finally, we'll get some action. I heard the nurse's voice on the intercom, asking Miranda to go to room 204.

While we waited, I made a blue monkey and a white monkey and a yellow tiger. My mom was now playing with chartreuse clay. I was getting a little tired of clay. It had been over an hour and still no aide. "I told you they don't come," she said sadly.

I went into the hallway, looking for anyone in scrubs. I stopped the first one I saw even though I didn't know her name. "Hi there, are you Miranda?"

"No, I'm not Miranda. I'm Debbie."

"Debbie, do you know where Miranda is? I need some help with my mom in room 204."

"Miranda's gone home for the day. She gets off work at three o'clock."

Miranda had already left work when that nurse paged her on the intercom! Didn't the nurse know that?

She probably did but only paged her to shut me up for another half hour.

I walked slowly back to the nurses' station. "Hi there," I said as brightly as I could, believing there was no point in showing anger. "I hear Miranda has gone home for the day, and my mom still needs to be changed and helped into bed. Can you tell me who her aide is now?"

"Oh, that would be Debbie."

God forbid Debbie to volunteer the information herself that she was supposed to be working in room 204! I shuffled off to find Debbie again, taking deep breaths to calm myself.

"Hi, Debbie. I guess you're the one I was looking for after all. My mom's been waiting over an hour and—"

Debbie cut me off. "I'm working my way down the hall. I'll get to her when I get to her."

My mother was still rolling the orange clay back and forth in her hands. "You're no help at all," she said to me sadly, and I agreed.

By the time Debbie sauntered into the room, all that was left of the clay color spectrum were the brown and the black. I placed the paper plates with the brightly colored clay blobs on Mom's tray table and left the room. Mom liked her privacy when she was having her diaper changed; although, occasionally, I did stick around to check her bedsore.

I felt absolutely helpless, worthless, and frustrated. I knew the nursing-home staff worked hard. I also knew my mother's life was not in danger. But should we really have to passively accept the fact that my mother would always have to wait at least an hour, and often longer than that, to have her diaper changed? How would her bedsore ever heal when it was constantly exposed to the bacteria in her diaper?

I sat out in the lobby and waited while Debbie got my mother onto the bed and changed her diaper. Somewhere in my mind, I knew I should be angry that the staff let her wait so long. Officially, per her doctor's orders, she was only to be out of bed for three to four hours per day. Two days earlier, they had left her up for over eight hours. On this day, when I first requested help with my mother, she had already been up for four hours. Even if all they had done was follow their own rules, an aide should have already come into her room to put her to bed.

I was too depressed to feel angry. The time I spent in the nursing home as a visitor no longer left me feeling entitled to anything. I felt like a perpetual beggar, pleading for crumbs of kindness. I kept searching for a tone of voice that would inspire a staff member to attend to my mother's needs.

I knew my mother's well-being rested largely on the whims of the staff, as well as the day-to-day vagaries of other patients. If another patient had a crisis or behaved violently toward the staff, then that patient would take precedence. If an aide's boyfriend had broken up with her the night before, talking to her girlfriends at work about it would take precedence. The government could legislate until they were blue in the face. They could impose sanctions for flagrant disregard of rules. And yet, for daily needs, we were at the mercy of these poorly paid men and women who worked at the nursing home.

There are things people will do for love. There are things people will do for money. The nursing home charged $6,800 per month for my mother to be there. At that time, she was a private-pay resident, so I knew exactly how much they were charging her. I hadn't expected this amount of money to buy love for her or even buy someone to care whether her fingernails were getting too long or her socks matched. Still, I had thought it would be enough money to buy the staff's attention— at least to see if my mother got to bed when she should, to change her diaper in less than thirty minutes, and to answer a call bell in a timely fashion. But it didn't.

As I sat in the lobby looking at the Halloween decorations, I felt demoralized. I had hoped my frequent, friendly presence in the nursing home would incline the staff to be kinder to my mother and perhaps, be a little more mindful of her. I realize now this had been a foolish hope. On my planned departure the following week, I would leave knowing she would be warm and safe. She would be cleaned probably twice a day. Because my mother's speech was so poor, it was unlikely that her requests for anything else would make their way to the staff's consciousness.

I had failed my mother—my tiny, fragile mom.

JOURNAL ENTRY 3-4

When I came back from lunch about four o'clock, my mom was awake but lying in bed. Several buzzers of different pitches were going off. Some buzzers meant a patient had pushed a call button for help. Other buzzers went off automatically when patients who were at risk of falling got out of their wheelchairs. If the wrong door was open, a buzzer alerted staff that a patient without outdoor privileges was trying to get out. The cacophony was extremely annoying.

Several TVs also blared. Poor old Lucy, one of the residents, was in the middle of the hall in her wheelchair, grabbing her crotch and grunting "bathroom." I don't know what illness Lucy had, but anyone could see that her hands were so crippled, they were bent completely backward. Obviously, the poor woman couldn't take herself to the bathroom.

Ethel, one of the few patients who could walk without a walker, came and vigorously pushed Lucy down the hall to the dining room. The floor nurse was only a few feet away, and she shouted for Ethel to take Lucy back to her room. Then an old guy walked down the hall with his walker, and the floor nurse yelled at him to go back to his room. Meanwhile, a woman named Lucille was in her wheelchair in the hall because her roommate, who was quite large, was having a shower; this maneuver required them to use the Hoyer lift, and there wasn't enough room for Lucille to sit in her wheelchair beside her own bed with the Hoyer lift in there. Lucille was also extremely hard of hearing, and it was obvious to me from her exasperated muttering that no one had explained to her why she had to sit in the hall.

I wondered, not for the first time, who had designed this building to be a nursing home. At first, I had assumed that the building was originally designed with a different purpose in mind and had been remodeled to be a nursing home. But someone told me that this building had been designed from the beginning to be a nursing home. Wheelchairs were in existence before this building was built. An extra four feet of width in the bathrooms, bedrooms, and sidewalks out front would have meant a world of difference to the people who lived here day in and day out. I couldn't tell you how many times I had jumped up to help a wheelchair patient maneuver their way into a room or even across the sidewalk because the dimensions were too narrow to easily navigate in a wheelchair.

It began to feel like bedlam to me. Ethel wheeled Lucy in the opposite direction, having apparently figured out that Lucy wanted the bathroom. Ethel told the aide, and the aide said Lucy would have to wait until Lucille's roommate finished her shower. Then June, an Alzheimer's patient who was very vocal at that time every day, began screeching like a giant bird of prey. She sometimes did it for hours at a time. Usually, I could tune her out, but now it was just one more aggravation. The noise and pain and confusion were almost more than I could bear—buzzers going off, Lucy grunting to go to the bathroom, the floor nurse yelling, Lucille spitting and cussing, and June screeching.

After the roommate was hoisted into bed, I knew
Lucille—who appeared to be in less need—would take
precedence over Lucy with her urgent need to go to the
bathroom; Lucy had no family, while Lucille's daughter
was a "big shot" in local government. If you don't think
the staff was aware of those details, you have not spent
much time in a nursing home. Lucille hadn't been there
very long, but her room was directly across the hall
from my mom's, so I had heard the way her daughter
spoke to the staff. I'd also seen how the staff, so far, had
immediately snapped to attention and given her what
she wanted—and I mean *immediately!*

I could also read the handwriting on the wall. I knew
there must have been only one aide on duty. By the time
she'd finished the roommate's shower and hoisted her
into bed, put Lucille back into bed, and then changed
Lucy—because, by then, Lucy would surely have gone
in her pants—it would be too late for her to get my mom
up and into her wheelchair for supper. It was already
five o'clock.

I had brought in some fresh clay for my mom, and we
amused ourselves playing with it—I figured it would be
a break from the boredom and good for her to exercise
her hands a little too. By now, most of the buzzers had
been shut off. Only one was buzzing away, but the TVs
were blaring at full volume, so conversation with my
mom was out of the question. I sang to Mom, silly
songs I usually sang for kids, inserting her name for any
name in the lyrics. My mom had never heard any of

these songs and thought I was making them up. She was very impressed.

Lucille's daughter had arrived. It turned out that her mother, who was very hard of hearing, had lost the headphones she wore most of the time, even to listen to television. The daughter stormed out of the room and down to the office area. When she came back, she was all sweetness and light. She told her mother not to worry, the nursing home would buy her a new set of headphones.

In the meantime, Lucy continued to propel herself up and down the hallway with her one good foot, asking everyone she met to take her to the bathroom. More buzzers went off. I was at my wits' end. The noise was fraying my nerves, my sympathy for poor old Lucy was flaying my heart, and my indignation at preferential treatment for the mother of a person with clout made me want to scream. No one would have heard me if I had.

I leaned over to my mom and spoke loudly into her ear. "Mom, I love you, but I'm tired, and I'm going to go now. I'll see you tomorrow." It was not quite six o'clock, but I couldn't take it anymore.

REPORTS FROM OTHERS

I met a young woman, Patricia, at a women's club meeting. While chatting with her, I learned that she had been a CNA in skilled nursing for five years until she went back to school in 2013. I asked her if she had any suggestions on how to get staff to answer a call bell. I was halfway hoping she would give me an incredulous look and tell me my mother must have been in a particularly lax facility. I wanted to hear that she had not encountered such lack of response in the facilities she'd worked in. Instead, she told me that, in her experience, the typical wait was one to one-and-a-half hours for a call bell to be answered.

My heart sank down to my toes. I asked, "Isn't there anything the family can do to get a quicker response?"

She gave me a big smile. "I loved going into the rooms of patients with personalized items on display, such as pictures, books, mementos, blankets, awards, military medals, and so on. I remember one guy who came through who was into baseball and he had tons of baseball awards on the wall. That helped me connect with him and remember that the person who loved baseball, was still inside that person in the wheelchair."

Patricia continued, "In that line of work, it is easy for someone to forget that their patient is a human being and there is love and joy still left in that person. It is too easy to just get caught up in getting them dressed and fed. I wish someone had trained me a little better so I could have been more sympathetic."

Andrea worked in several care facilities in Wisconsin in more than one role. She was able to describe for me what care was given in different types of long-term care facilities. She is now an activities director, but she worked for eight years as a CNA. She told me that when she was an aide in a physical rehabilitation facility, their goal was to respond to a call button within ten minutes. But as a CNA in a skilled nursing facility for six years, she learned that the call button lights there elicited no response. As she explained, "You [the visitor] can't make assumptions that something will just happen. You have to physically go and get the help you need. The call light is not going to get it done. But do it in a way that is not accusing or condemning because those CNAs are working their tails off."

Andrea took it a step further and told me about a woman she had known a long time. This woman had been a dependable and enthusiastic volunteer at one nursing home. When this long-time volunteer needed to be in a long-term care facility herself as a resident, Andrea assumed that the staff, who knew her as the "Music Lady," would be extremely responsive to any reasonable requests she made. Andrea's expectations were dashed when she visited her friend and discovered that responses to her call button took as long as they did for anyone else.

I asked if there would be any benefit to bringing cookies or other food treats to the staff. This had been suggested to my sister and me by the elder law attorney we consulted, and we had followed this advice without any evident benefit. Andrea shrugged off this suggestion. "The problem is that the CNAs are just desperately trying to get everyone taken care of. There is no way, apart from better staffing, that you are going to get better response times." She was adamant that family members should not give money to a staff member in hopes of better service. "The whole thing about giving money is a huge no-no. Shame on them for accepting money because they should never ever accept money from a patient. Unfortunately, there is no way to bribe for more attention. It was really stressed at my facility—you cannot accept a cash gift, partly because the giver can later claim the money was stolen."

Betty, also a former CNA, said, "The bigger the patient was in size, the more likely we were told not to answer their call button to get them to the toilet. We were told to let them soil themselves because it was less time consuming to eventually change a diaper than to hoist the person out of bed, put them on the toilet, stand there in case they lost their balance, and then help them back into the bed again."

FOR THE RECORD

The Iowa Department of Inspections and Appeals has actually mandated that nursing-home staff must answer call buttons within fifteen minutes.[13] As far as I know, Iowa is the only state to date to have enacted a regulation specifically mandating an acceptable time to answer a call bell in a nursing home.

TIPS

- Bring in photos and memorabilia from your loved one's life prior to their residence in the nursing home. Post these on the door, the wall, or anywhere the staff can't miss them.
- Decorate the room and the door for seasons and holidays. This will lift the spirits of the resident and provide an easy topic of conversation for any aides or visitors. Digital photo frames are excellent.
- Don't wait for the call button to be answered. Go find a staff person and bring the need to their attention, but do it in a way that is not accusatory or condemning. Be mindful that most CNAs are working very hard for very low pay.
- Don't expect any better response by bringing in cookies or treats.
- Avoid giving a cash gift to a staff member.

CHAPTER 4
Swallowing Issues

"Hungry," my mother croaked. She said this several times each day, and it broke my heart. I'd already explained to her many times the consequences for her if she tried to eat normal food again. I explained again. "Mom, the muscles in your throat are still not very strong from your stroke. That is why you have trouble swallowing. If you eat something, there is a chance it won't go down your throat to your stomach, but instead it will go down into your lungs. This can cause you to get pneumonia. You could die."

"How many?"

"How many what?"

"How many days without food?" It was hard for her to put so many words together. Her enunciation was not good, but I finally understood her question.

I calculated in my head. "More than fifty."

She was quiet for a while, considering. "Jesus only went forty."

"Mom." I stared deep into her eyes, trying to gauge if she had enough mental competency to fully understand the risks. "Mom, do you want to take the chance you might die? Do you understand that if they take out the feeding tube, you might die?"

"Yeth," she said with conviction. It then took a while for her to get the words out, and I had to guess at most of them. "I am not afraid to die. I will never get better if I don't eat."

The conversation that followed was the closest we'd ever had to a heart-to-heart. My mother said she'd had a good, long life without being sick until that year. She said her soul was saved by Jesus, and so she did not fear death because death would mean going to heaven. Of course, between her brain damage and her speech difficulties, this meaning did not come out smoothly. It came in spurts and sputters. She became irritated with herself. I guessed at what she was trying to say and said it back to her for confirmation or modification. She was absolutely exhausted from the effort and finally fell asleep.

I told Jenny about Mom's decision. Jenny called Dr. Adam's office and left a message, saying our mom wanted the feeding tube removed and was willing to assume the risk.

JOURNAL ENTRY 4-2

I looked down at my tiny mother in her bed, bundled up with a red cape draping her head and shoulders, pink velour mittens on her hands, and a blue blanket pulled up to her chin. Jenny and I had left her in her Geri chair in the lobby near the nurses' station while we went out to lunch and visited our aunt Molly. Before we left, we'd told her floor nurse we'd left Mom in the lobby and hoped someone would check on her while we were gone.

When we walked into the lobby at four o'clock, we were dismayed to find her still sitting where we'd left her.

"I'm cold!" she said plaintively. I took her hands in mine—they were indeed terribly cold. It wasn't a bitterly cold day, and she was fully dressed, but when the door to the lobby opened for visitors to come and go, it let in the fresh air and wind.

We hustled our mom to her room. It was the first time Jenny and I had put her in bed on our own without waiting for a staff person. We each supported her under an arm. From the wheelchair, we half dragged her to the exact spot where she needed to plant her butt so her body would conform comfortably when the head of the bed was raised. I was terrified we might somehow damage her with our clumsiness, but we were desperate to get her warm. As soon as we got her into the bed, we piled on some blankets. She complained her hands were cold, so we put mittens on her. I wished we'd had a camera to take her picture because she looked like one of those dried apple dolls you see at craft shows.

JOURNAL ENTRY 4-3

For Halloween, my sister had found a bright orange T-shirt that said, "Don't Make Me Scare You." She coached our mom to say "Boo!" whenever someone commented on her shirt. It was so cute the way she would say "Boo!" in such a tiny voice. I found myself falling more in love with my little mother. She was so fragile and cute sometimes, especially when her hair was unbrushed and sticking up on top of her head like a little troll doll.

Again, I had to search a long time for the control for my mom's bed, which I finally found under the mattress. I didn't think the staff did this to be mean or obnoxious. Instead, I believed (and still believe) it was the result of complete indifference.

JOURNAL ENTRY 4-4

I marked this day on the calendar as the day Mom started eating again even though she still had the feeding tube. The speech pathologist had coached her about tucking her chin when she swallowed. Mom promised she would do this. She began with mashed potatoes with butter on them, and although she coughed a little bit, she did okay overall.

I've had no children, but that day, I felt as I imagine a mother would, watching her child dive into a pool for the first time. My heart went out to her as she performed this daring feat—putting food into her mouth. I couldn't help her with it; she had to swallow for herself. I felt so helpless.

JOURNAL ENTRY 4-5

Jenny went back home yesterday. I missed her. I missed having someone to talk with about Mom.

I went out to lunch, and when I came back, I placed my lips near Mom's ear. "I love you, Monkey Mom," I said loudly. And I meant it. I'd said this to her probably a dozen times since her stroke, and she had never once said it back to me. But I was finding that I didn't need her to reciprocate. I wished she would, but whether she did or not, the spigot had been turned to the open position, and love continued to flow out of me and into her. I wondered, not for the first time, if this love I felt for her was somehow God loving her through me, that I was only a conduit and not really an active part in this flow of love. I had been praying to God to keep sending her His love through me or any other conduit.

Oh my God, how can I possibly leave her? I was distraught at the thought of leaving her to fend for herself as helpless as she was.

I thought of the book *The Little Prince* and the main character who fears for his rose because she is defenseless, with only three thorns, even though she thinks her thorns make her fierce. The little prince protects her by placing a glass jar over her at night.

My rose did not even have thorns, and her voice was too weak to yell for help. She really was defenseless.

JOURNAL ENTRY 4-6

I'd been back in Wisconsin for two weeks.

On this day, when I got home, there was a message on the phone from my mom. Her roommate's daughter, Connie, had called me on her cellphone and then coached my mom through the phone message. "Say, 'Hi Ruthie,'" I heard in the background. And then my little mom's voice said, "Hi, Ruthie." That was the whole message, but it was enough for me to know she was okay and Connie was looking out for her, at least a little. I was extremely grateful. I was as content as was possible, being one thousand miles away from Mom.

JOURNAL ENTRY 4-7

My sister returned to see Mom and had a lot to report. Our mother had been "acting up" with the staff. She had been combative and resisted them when they tried to dress and undress her. They were giving her risperidone again to make her more placid. Of course, no one had *called* either of us to tell us this was going on. I had no idea why this was happening. I was both relieved and angry she was on risperidone again. I had written a letter to Dr. Adams a few months ago, asking him to please keep Mom on the risperidone as I had seen a marked improvement in her overall behavior while she had been on it. He had declined to refill the prescription at that time.

She still had the feeding tube in her stomach, but they were not feeding her that way right now. The machine that pumped the artificial food through her feeding tube was shut off. I guessed they were testing to see how she would do eating by mouth. It was disturbing to me that Mom was coughing quite a bit when she ate. Each time she coughed while eating a particular food, she decided it was the specific food item that was causing her to cough. She then would refuse to eat that food item again. This was quite problematic. With the narrow categories of foods she was willing to eat, foods they served at the nursing home, and foods that had now caused her to cough, she was limited to a very small menu of food items.

JOURNAL ENTRY 4-8

They took the feeding tube out of my mom today. At least, I think they did. Jenny called the nursing home yesterday to ask how Mom was doing, and the nurse made an offhand comment. "Oh, by the way, your mom is going to the hospital tomorrow to have her feeding tube removed."

I couldn't call Mom on the phone to tell her about the procedure because she didn't have a phone. I could only hope that a staff member had taken the time to tell her about it, reassure her it would be a very quick procedure, and inform her she would return to the nursing home that same day. I had no way of finding out.

Oh good, Jenny just called. Mom was back at the nursing home. The feeding-tube removal went off without a hitch. I hoped Mom understood what was going on.

The *important* thing to me about removing the tube was that Jenny could stop feeling guilty about it. Ever since Mom had been able to let us know that she preferred to die and wished we had let her do so on Labor Day, Jenny had been feeling guilty; it was she who had agreed to the feeding tube placement. I had told my sister at least a dozen times that she shouldn't feel guilty and that I had also agreed to the procedure. I reminded her we had no way of knowing then that Mom would have preferred to die. I finally gave up when I realized this wasn't a guilt from which I could possibly absolve her.

Jenny wished desperately to place Mom back where she had been before we had interfered by calling the neighbor to rescue her and then interfered further by agreeing to the feeding tube. Now that the tube was removed and we had the advance medical directive tattooed on our hearts, we would be ready if anyone suggested that procedure again. We now knew to say no. I was really happy for Jenny that the feeding tube was out.

Although the feeding tube had been removed, Mom still was not allowed to eat or drink normally. A packet of thickener had to be mixed into any liquid, including hot tea and plain water, before Mom could drink it. Food items had to be pureed. According to the staff, she was still at risk of aspirating food or water into her lungs, which could cause pneumonia.

Despite instructions from the floor nurse and the speech therapist, it was not unusual for me to walk into Mom's room and find a pitcher of water with a glass on her tray table. Aides still occasionally delivered food to her that was not pureed. When I told the aide who had delivered the water or nonpureed food to my mother that this was not allowed, the answer was always the same—a blank look. The floor nurse had posted a sign over my mother's bed with a warning, but it simply said NPO, an acronym for the Latin words *nil per os,* which translates as "nothing by mouth." I honestly had my doubts whether any of the aides understood this warning.

FOR THE RECORD

There are about four hundred fifty thousand Americans living with nourishment from feeding tubes. Many live at home in nonmedical settings and are able to care for the equipment and choose their own formula or food.[14] Common reasons for placement of a feeding tube include trouble swallowing for whatever reason; cancer impacting the head or neck muscles; chronic loss of appetite due to severe illness; or treatment for that illness.[15]

There are three main types of feeding tubes named according to their location on the body. A feeding tube that is inserted into the nose is called a "nasogastric tube" and does not require surgery for placement or removal. "Gastric tubes" can only be placed during surgery, and they go directly into the stomach. These can be permanent or temporary. "Jejunostomy tubes," also placed during surgery, bypass the stomach and go directly into the small intestine.[16]

Patients and their loved ones should be fully informed of the risks and benefits of feeding tubes before one is placed. Although this decision can sometimes be easy, there are situations where the decision becomes more difficult, such as when the patient has a living will that specifies they never want to use a feeding tube. In some of these cases, however, the medical professionals or the family or both may think there is a chance the patient will recover if fed through a feeding tube to keep nutrition and hydration flowing. Still, a feeding tube is not always the right choice.

When it is time to transition from dependence on a feeding tube to eating food by mouth, there should be a gradual weaning off from the feeding tube. During this time, the patient will continue to receive some feeding tube nutrition but will increase intake of food by mouth. If weight can be maintained for at least two weeks without use of the feeding tube, then the feeding tube can be removed.[17]

SIDE NOTE: Risperidone is used to treat people with bipolar disorder, schizophrenia, and other disorders. Once my mother had her first TIA, she was intermittently prescribed risperidone. My sister and I saw a dramatic improvement in her demeanor and implored the nursing-home staff and her doctor—both in writing and in person—to keep her on risperidone. They always refused. We both thought it was because they were worried she would become addicted to it, but since she was eighty-nine years old, we believed the benefits would outweigh the risk of addiction or dependence.

TIPS

- Don't count on the staff to give your loved one the optimal feeding formula. Do some research yourself. There are a variety of formulas. When a friend who is a registered dietician (RD) visited my mother in the nursing home, she was appalled that they were not giving her a high protein formula. According to the RD, my mother desperately needed all the protein she could get to help heal her bedsores.

- Continue dental care, even if your loved one is not eating or drinking anything by mouth. Teeth, gums, and tongue should be brushed daily.[18]

- Keep an eye out for skin problems such as redness or irritation at the feeding-tube entry site.

- Be aware that diarrhea or constipation can be a side effect of the feeding tube.

- Visit The Feeding Tube Awareness Foundation's website—https://www.feedingtubeawareness.org/.http Their primary audience is parents of children with feeding tubes, but they provide a wealth of information also useful for adults on feeding tubes.

- Don't assume all aides can read English fluently. Post pictures of water near your loved one and write "no" or a big "X" through them. It is worth a try.

CHAPTER 5
Baths

JOURNAL ENTRY 5-1

The aides came to give my mother her weekly bath tonight. Mom, who had taken a bath in a bathtub every day of her life in her own home, absolutely hated showers in the nursing home. For one thing, they put her in a plastic sling chair, which, because she was short, threw her off-balance so she didn't feel supported. Her feet did not touch the ground when she sat naked and wet in the large, tiled shower room.

This was how they gave her a shower: they took off her clothes, and then they sprayed her down. The water couldn't be warmer than lukewarm because they didn't want to risk damaging old and fragile skin with hot water. She was soaped, then rinsed with another spray. Then the aides went to get a towel while my mother sat in her plastic chair, soaking wet and shivering. They dried her, put on her nightgown, wheeled her back to her room, and put her to bed with wet hair.

Each patient had a weekly shower time. My mother's was Friday night. This was a particularly inauspicious time slot for two reasons: First, they took her late in the evening, often after she had already fallen asleep, so they had to wake her up. Second, the hairdresser only came to the nursing home on Thursdays, so my mom would have her hair fixed on Thursdays only to have it ruined on Fridays.

My mother had always been ridiculously vain about her hair; she had faithfully visited the hairdresser weekly for as long as I could remember. She would have it permed, teased, sprayed, and tinted. She always wore a rain bonnet when she went outside to keep her hair from being mussed by the elements—whether it was raining or not. She slept on a satin pillow with a satin hair wrap to keep her hair in place.

So, although I'd always been a wash-and-wear kind of girl, I could sympathize with my mom. She hated to have her hair looking horrible for five days out of seven when it could have been prevented. Yes, it was vanity. She was eighty-nine and in a nursing home. Whom did she think she was impressing? Regardless, I hoped changing the shower schedule would make her a little happier.

This is all to explain that both Jenny and I had already gone to the nursing staff to request a change in my mother's shower schedule. We also knew she had refused a shower on more than one occasion. My sister and I had even refused the shower on her behalf if she really didn't want to have it. Our request for a schedule change had always been denied.

Today when my mother protested her shower, the aide very kindly said she could give my mother a sponge bath in her bed instead. My mother and sister were very grateful. The director of nursing happened to poke her head in while the aide was retrieving whatever she needed for my mom's sponge bath. Jenny related this act of kindness to the director of nursing who said, "Oh, she can always get a sponge bath instead of a shower. We can put it on her care checklist inside her closet door."

Jenny said, "That sounds great, but she doesn't have any sort of checklist inside her closet door."

The nurse bustled over to Mom's closet, insisting, "Oh, of course she does. *Every* patient does. The checklist shows whether the patient needs help with certain things, wears a hearing aid, wears glasses, whether the family or the nursing home does the laundry, and so on." When she flung open Mom's closet door with a flourish to show my sister, there was no checklist! Jenny had never seen a checklist there and neither had I. The nurse was the only one surprised not to see one.

The nurse retrieved a checklist form, filled it out, and posted it on the inside of my mother's closet door. There was finally a written request for my mother to be given a sponge bath instead of a shower—after she had endured five months of Friday night showers!

First, it made me crazy to learn there had been a *choice* all along. How many showers had my mom endured since September without knowing she could have asked for a sponge bath? Second, how could it be that she had been there for five months and not a single staff person noticed she did not have this checklist that supposedly every patient had? As cynical as I had already become about this facility, I wondered how much the staff would pay attention to the checklist now that she had one. Having for so long not noticed its absence, would any staff notice its presence and abide by her requests?

I was beyond screaming or crying. I hurt for Mom. I also worried about my own future self who may land in a nursing home someday. How would I fare without a daughter to advocate for me? We were trying as hard as we could, but my sister and I had often been unsuccessful in improving our mom's life here.

REPORTS FROM OTHERS

When I interviewed Samantha about her husband's tenure in a nursing home, she brought up the issue of bathing. "He hated getting a shower because they were so rough with him. And they *never* said he could have had a sponge bath instead. I thought the shower was required." Two years after his death, her bitterness over this was palpable.

Claire Johnson was similarly outraged, but it was at the *lack* of bathing for her mother. "They didn't give her baths. She was scheduled to have them on Tuesday and

Friday. If she missed one due to a doctor's visit or lack of staffing, they made her wait until her next scheduled one. Yet, it was actually part of her care plan to have showers twice a week." When her mother was moved to a second facility, the bathing issue got even worse. "They didn't give her a bath for two weeks. The nursing home said they had given her a bath on such and such day, yet I had been there all day that day and they had not given her a bath. They outright lied about it. Then she finally had a shower, and it was given by a man, which totally freaked my mother out."

Betty, a former CNA in North Carolina, remembered, "All the residents where I was a CNA had no family that ever visited, and we were understaffed. They didn't have enough equipment, so the one shower chair would be used by multiple people without cleaning it between people. Patients would get showers once a week if they were lucky."

FOR THE RECORD

"Should nursing home residents be forced to take showers?" was the headline in a March 20, 2013, article in the *Sarasota Herald-Tribune*.[19] A year earlier, a patient in a nursing home, Mary Ware, had died while being forcibly showered. Although the nursing home was ultimately absolved of wrongdoing, this investigation helped shine a light on an issue I had thought was a struggle only for my family. Indeed, during roughly the same time period as my tiny mom was fighting against being forcibly showered, Philip D. Sloane, a medical professor at the University of North Carolina, was leading a national movement to halt nursing homes from forcing residents to be showered against their will.

Dr. Sloane conducted research on bathing techniques in nine nursing homes in Oregon and six in North Carolina. He reported the positive effects of bed baths: "Agitation was down, skin condition actually improved, and there was no change in bacterial counts from those taken before the study." For patients with dementia who were switched to in-bed bathing, aggressive incidents during bathing declined by 60 percent.[20]

On the other side of the bathing coin were nursing-home residents who felt they were not given showers or bathed frequently enough. The University of Minnesota School of Public Health lists on its website specific states with regulations that mandate minimum bathing. Some states, such as Virginia and Indiana, require a minimum of two per week. New Jersey only requires one bath per week.[21]

TIPS

- Do not assume that a shower—as opposed to a bed bath—is required by law. It is not.
- Get a copy of Dr. Sloane's video if the staff do not give your loved one a bed bath, and the resident prefers a bed bath over a shower. Print his research article and give it, along with the video, to the director of nursing. A copy of the video *Bathing Without a Battle*© can be ordered on the website, https://bathingwithoutabattle.unc.edu/ or via email message to info@bathingwithoutabattle.unc.edu.

CHAPTER 6
Visiting

I decided I couldn't hold a job back home in Wisconsin and still travel to visit my mom as much as I wanted to in New Jersey. I was sure Mom didn't have much time left. I only had one mother, and she was only going to die once. I found myself flooded with a fierce love for her as well as a desire to protect and comfort her as much as possible until her death. And if I could do anything to give her joy and pleasure while she was dying, that would be an added benefit. I told Luke, my husband, my decision, and he readily agreed.

I knew there were people who would think badly of me for this decision. Some would say to themselves, "Her mother is in a nursing home, so why does she think she needs to visit her mom every day?" I also knew there were people who would think badly of me because I hadn't rearranged my life a year ago to be geographically closer to my mother. There was probably another faction, those who would believe I was wicked, ungrateful, lazy, self-centered, and more not to have my mother live in my own home. I was well aware of these points of view because many people had already shared their unsolicited opinions with me!

The bottom line was that I was tired of feeling like I had been cheating on my job whenever I ran off to see my mom. I also felt rushed the whole time I was home, trying to catch up on my job, church roles, and volunteer commitments. It had been a year of feeling I had to make every minute count. I couldn't hang out for an afternoon with a friend because I had to go to a meeting, write a paper, meet with a donor, or send out email announcements.

I was also tired of feeling as though I was rushing in and out of my mom's life. It was obvious she was slower in every respect. It took her nearly an hour to eat one scoop of mashed potatoes and a cup of pudding. It took at least a minute for her to respond with a yes or no answer to a simple question. Her pace had slowed, and I wanted enough time for me to adjust to *her* speed while she died.

I perused Craigslist for sublets. They were more expensive than I had guessed, but I was not deterred. Now that I had this plan, I was on fire to make it happen. I called three places and visited one. The one that interested me most didn't return my call. We were to leave for home the next day, but I remained confident that something would turn up.

JOURNAL ENTRY 6-2

Because I had been here for an extended period, my visits to my mom had become more relaxed. I sought out creative ways to spend time with her. Not solely to entertain her, but also, I hoped, to aid in her recuperation. Her speech therapist told us it was essential we encourage Mom to talk more. Mom was reluctant to initiate speech because she became very frustrated when she couldn't find the right words. It seemed I was always trying to get her to talk!

After lunch today, I took Mom outside. I had brought a picture book with large, colorful pictures of dogs. Dogs herding sheep, playing with kittens, and swimming—these were all pictures I used to engage Mom in conversation.

After supper, I asked the aide to put her to bed, and I happened to glance at my watch when I made the request. It was a little before six o'clock. The aide came at 6:30 p.m., which hadn't been a bad response interval for the nursing home. I told Mom at 6:30 p.m. that I was leaving, and she asked me not to go. She said she'd been having such a nice time with me and she hated for it to end. It was the first time she had ever expressed such a feeling to me. Of course, I stayed.

I sang to her even though she had her hearing aids out. Often, when I sang to her, I stopped and paused where a word should have been to encourage her to say the missing word. She usually complied with this. Sometimes, she tapped her finger along with the beat. But that night, she actually tried to sing along with the melody. Her voice was totally off the correct pitch, but I was thrilled by her effort. When I sang "It Had To Be You," it was all I could do not to laugh out loud because she sounded so much like my little dog Pixie. Pixie howled when I played the clarinet, and here was Mom warbling *youuuuuuu* just like my little dog. It was delightful! To paraphrase from *My Fair Lady,* I could have sung all night.

JOURNAL ENTRY 6-3

Although I had sung to my mom many times, I always looked longingly at the piano in the nursing home's dining room. I had started piano lessons when I was eight years old and the piano was a second skin for me. I wasn't sure if I would violate a rule if I played it, but today, I got up my courage and asked the person in charge of the dining room if I could play the piano during lunch. I got a big smile and an enthusiastic yes.

I hustled back to Mom's room and grabbed my copy of *Reader's Digest Family Songbook*. I settled Mom into a chair with her lunch and a plastic spoon in her hand and walked over to the piano. It wasn't too badly out of tune, and all the keys, except one, were in working condition. Ah, it felt so good to be rippling my hands across the keyboard again, playing songs that were the aural equivalent of roast chicken and gravy. A few residents sang along between bites of food. I got a hearty round of applause when I finished. My mother, however, was not pleased.

I was beaming when I reclaimed my seat next to her. "Mom, how did you like the music?"

"Hmpf" was all I got out of her. But I already knew I'd be playing the piano in the dining room again soon.

JOURNAL ENTRY 6-4

The mother of someone I once dated, a guy named Tony, was a resident at Pineville when my mom was there. His mother had dementia, but she liked to chat. Tony lived in the same town as the nursing home, but he never visited his mother. In fact, he actually paid someone else to visit his mom twice a week.

I know from experience that most people, like Tony, dislike visiting nursing homes. There are probably many different reasons why people have this feeling, but I figured one may have been an awkward sense of not knowing what to say or do. In hopes that my experience may help others, I am sharing the approach I developed after visiting my mother's nursing home for over a year.

Whenever I entered the nursing home, there were usually several residents sitting in the lobby in their wheelchairs, just hoping for a little bit of diversion in their day. The UPS delivery man, the mail man, and an ambulance were all a welcome variety even if the visit was an impersonal one. A visitor with a friendly dog was welcome, and even more so, a visitor who greeted them by name. Best of all was any visitor who had come especially to see them.

I greeted the residents I knew by name. Sometimes, I stopped to say something I hoped was pleasant. I had often agonized over what would be appropriate to say to someone who hadn't left the nursing home in months, or even years, and would probably never leave it again. Was it fair to mention the weather or traffic to people who never got outside? Did it only remind them of the simplest parts of life they were cut away from? I tried hard to be conversational and friendly, but offering only general observations such as weather, holidays and more.

I frequently pushed people down the hall in their wheelchairs. I had long refrained from doing this unless they were extremely distressed because I figured the exercise from wheeling the chair themselves was good for them. But I soon decided I'd routinely stop and ask if people would like a push. Occasionally they would say no, but they were often extremely grateful.

If Mom's roommate was in trouble in the bathroom, I'd hurry down the hall and ask a staff person to come help her. If it was something small I could do myself—opening a door, getting a spoon, finding a bib, opening a milk carton—I'd do those for anybody. As a person with full use of my limbs and speech, I found myself with a power the residents didn't have: to physically go and find a staff person and make myself understood.

Residents were in the nursing home for many reasons. Some had cancer while others had Alzheimer's. Some, like my mom, were residents because of a stroke. A great number of them had memory problems and speech issues. Although I didn't know the diagnoses of most of the patients, it was obvious that, like my mother, they could not put together a declarative sentence such as, "I love strawberries, but I can't eat these because they are too big to fit on the spoon." So if I saw someone at my mother's dining room table ignoring their strawberries, I'd try asking questions. "Are you still hungry?" "Do you like strawberries?" "Is there something wrong with those strawberries?" Maybe they were too cold to eat or had begun to spoil. "Are you having trouble eating them?" Maybe they needed to be cut into smaller pieces. "Would you rather have pudding?"

I could spare three or four minutes with Dottie at the lunch table to help her express her food preferences. Dottie still had enough of her mind to know she liked strawberries, but she couldn't eat them because they kept rolling off her spoon; she didn't have enough speech to communicate this to a staff person. Added to this was another layer of communication difficulties— many of the staff spoke English very poorly. My ability to move between these two worlds began to feel like a power of near-mythic proportions. It wasn't the end of the world if Dottie had to sit there and look at her juicy red strawberries and not eat them, but it was a small kindness I could offer her, to grab a knife and fork and cut those berries up into smaller pieces.

REPORTS FROM OTHERS

My sister and I had often speculated whether our mom was getting less attention from the nursing-home staff because they knew we would be there. We often took up the slack and did things like brush her hair, clean her glasses, cut her nails, bring her pudding, and peel her bananas. We wondered if perhaps she would have received more attention from the staff had we visited less often. So I posed this question to my interviewees.

Sue Roberts, a former marketing director for a nursing home, said, "Absolutely. The staff knows whether a patient is getting a lot of visitors or not. And they definitely get treated better if they do have a lot of visitors." So my sister and I had our answer!

Martha had worked in the laundry room of a nursing home until they were so short of CNAs that they asked her to be an aide. "There was a blind person there, and they didn't even tell him where his food was on the table or on his plate. The only time they really paid attention to a patient was when the family was there. Those who only got one visit per month didn't get attention the rest of the time." Martha added, "When I brought a problem to the administration, they didn't want to hear it." She was so disgusted by the standard of care, she quit after a few months.

Samantha advised, "You have to be there [as a visitor] every day. I often wonder what would happen if I couldn't visit every day. After you have been there every day for several weeks, then they know that you are going to be there. I think it makes a big difference in how they deal with the patient."

FOR THE RECORD

More than 50 percent of the residents in nursing homes have no close relative and 46 percent have no living children. That's according to the National Center for Health Statistics (NCHS). It is also estimated that 60 percent of nursing-home residents never have visitors.[22]

If you are reading this book, chances are excellent that you will visit your loved ones in the nursing home! Robyn Grant, director of public policy and advocacy for the National Consumer Voice for Quality Long-Term Care, advised, "The number one thing to do is to visit as many times, and at different times, as possible. Vary the time of day that you go in."[23] This will benefit your loved one because you will be able to see for yourself interaction with staff, quality of food, and grooming (or lack thereof). You'll be able to check for bedsores and quickly spot whether glasses or hearing aids are missing.

Remember that even if your loved one is in relatively good health and not suffering with an infectious disease, someone else in the facility may be! On the other hand, you yourself may be harboring an infection that won't manifest itself for another day. You should wash your hands when you arrive and avoid visiting a long-term care facility altogether if you know you are sick. Wash your hands before you leave.[24]

TIPS

- Be at the nursing home in person as often as you can. You don't have to spend all day there; even a half-hour visit will make a difference in how the staff treats your loved one.

- Try to be aware of the other residents you encounter even though your focus will be on your loved one during the visit. Roommates should be respected—knock before entering the room. Ask permission before you turn the television volume down or off. Remember that other residents are people, too, and would appreciate a friendly greeting from you in the hall or common areas.
- Visit in the afternoon, as mornings are usually more hectic than afternoons. It would generally be preferable to visit in the afternoon.
- Bring something with you for a conversation starter, such as a local newspaper or a picture album.
- Help your loved one send a card or letter to a friend or relative. If they have trouble with their penmanship, you can do the writing for them. Bring stationery or cards, then put the postage on and mail it for them.
- Don't worry about bringing a gift. Keep in mind, there are space limitations in the residents' rooms.

CHAPTER 7
Hearing Aids and Glasses

Alta, a woman from my mother's church who was nearly as old as my mom, called Jenny today to ask if she knew that Mom's glasses had been lost. When Alta had visited the previous week, Mom hadn't had them then either. Jenny thanked her for her kindness in letting her know.

When Jenny called the nursing home, the social worker, Mindy, wasn't sure when the optometrist would visit again, but she assured Jenny she would put Mom's name on the patient list for the next time. Mindy couldn't be bothered to check her computer, file cabinet, or calendar to see when the optometrist was coming. Well, it didn't matter; he'd get there when he got there.

Jenny called me with this information. Of course, we were frustrated. Neither of us had been to Pineville for a month. Mom had had her glasses the day I left, but how long had they been missing? I had suggested last fall that we get Mom a backup pair of glasses from her regular optometrist for a situation like this. Jenny had agreed it was a good idea and called the optometrist, but he refused to make Mom another pair of glasses without seeing her in his office. Even when Jenny had explained the situation—the nursing home, wheelchair, and stroke—he remained unmoved. He had his rules. He didn't clarify whether they were professional rules, personal rules, or state rules, but now my mom would pay the price.

JOURNAL ENTRY 7-2

Mom's minister called Jenny today. When Jenny saw Mom's area code on her caller ID, she was worried. Then, when the caller turned out to be Mom's minister, she immediately assumed the worst. Instead, he explained he had his cell phone with him in the nursing home and thought he would do us a kindness by putting Mom on the phone with Jenny.

Sadly, Jenny was unable to understand what our mother was trying to say. Jenny tried asking yes-and-no questions, but she couldn't understand Mom's responses to those either. Jenny tried her best to tell Mom she was on the list to get new glasses, but she couldn't tell if Mom understood.

We wondered if she'd had another stroke and if she was still getting speech therapy. We wouldn't have blamed the powers that be if they had discontinued it, but without Jenny or me there to work with her, we wondered how much she would try to talk.

JOURNAL ENTRY 7-3

Juanita called Jenny to tell her the optometrist was at the nursing home. Juanita just happened to be there, and she saw him setting up in the dining room. She also took the liberty, thank goodness, of going to check whether Mom's name was on the list of residents to be seen. It wasn't, so Juanita was calling to ask if Jenny wanted Mom's eyes examined.

This was extremely frustrating because the social worker had assured Jenny just last week that she would put Mom's name on the list to see the optometrist. Jenny begged Juanita to get Mom in to see the optometrist while he was there. Juanita said she would do her best.

JOURNAL ENTRY 7-4

Jenny went to visit our mom for the Fourth of July holiday. It turned out Mom *could* talk, but the staff just hadn't been taking enough time for her to formulate a response. Jenny said there was a delay between when you asked Mom a question and when she answered, but she was able to answer. You just had to have a lot of patience. Also, Mom didn't voluntarily speak without prompting; you had to solicit a response with a question.

Mom still didn't have her new glasses, so Jenny went to the dollar store and bought several pairs of reading glasses for Mom to try. They wouldn't replace the prescription for her nearsightedness, but they should enhance her ability to read. Mom was incapable, or unwilling, of providing feedback as to which of the pairs most improved her vision.

We found out they had lost one of her hearing aids too. We had no idea when this happened. She definitely had them when I'd visited four months ago.

JOURNAL ENTRY 7-5

After Mom fell asleep, I looked for her glasses and found the six pairs of reading glasses, evidently the ones Jenny bought at the dollar store. There was no pair with prescription bifocal lenses. I called Jenny, who sighed and said she'd tried to follow up on it, but the optical store said they wouldn't make the glasses until they had received payment. Jenny was eager to pay, but no one had sent her a bill.

"Give me the address," I said as calmly as I could manage, "and I'll go pay for them."

I could hear Jenny rummaging to find the paperwork. "Oh my God," she sputtered when she'd found it, "it's some place on the other side of Philadelphia. Why on earth do they use a place so far away? Are the optometrists in the Pineville area *too busy* to go to the nursing home?"

Just because I was already in a bad mood, I decided to also ask about the hearing aids. Jenny explained, "The nursing home still says it isn't their fault they were lost. They say they were lost in the hospital last February. Therefore, the nursing home won't pay the deductible on the insurance to replace them." For more on that hospital visit, see chapter 10.

That made me explode. "*No way* did the hospital lose them! I didn't even take the hearing aids to the hospital! They'd been here, in her room, when I came and got her glasses and hair brush. They were not sent with her when she was shipped to the hospital, and I didn't take them there. Besides, how much *is* the damn deductible anyway? Just tell me, and I'll pay it. This is so ridiculous, for Mom to be lying here day after day unable to see anything or hear anything."

Jenny admitted she didn't know the deductible amount, but she promised to find out.

JOURNAL ENTRY 7-6

An amazing thing happened today. Diana, Mom's floor nurse for the day shift today, bustled up to me and asked about Mom's hearing aids. She said, "See, the thing is, the nursing home isn't going to pay the deductible if they were lost at the hospital."

I usually bent over backward to be polite and deferential to the staff who took care of my mom. This time, I'd had it with the hearing aid business. I explained to her, in no uncertain terms, that my mom *never had* her hearing aids at the hospital, so they could not have been lost there. I asked *her* how much the deductible was. She didn't know either and scurried away to find out.

An hour later, Diana poked her head into my mom's room. "I wanted to let you know the nursing home has decided to pay the deductible on your mother's hearing aids. But this is the last time we're going to do that."

"Well that's great!" I said, leaping to my feet. "That is really great. Do you know how long it will take?"

"I'm not sure when they will get here, but I'll let you know," she promised.

"Oh, Diana, listen. Would it be possible for Mom to get one of those attachment things on her hearing aids like I see on other patients' hearing aids? Somehow, they get these strings attached to the hearing aids and there are clips on the ends of the strings. Then you can clip the strings to their clothing so the hearing aids won't get lost."

"Sure thing, I'll make a note of that."

JOURNAL ENTRY 7-7

The lady from the audiology clinic showed up to make impressions of Mom's ears. I asked *her* about the strings with the clips on them, but she acted like she had never in her life heard of such a thing. I hurried down the hall until I found another patient with these strings and showed them to her. She called her boss and described them to him.

"Okay," she told me, "if you get the alligator clips for the ends of the string, I'll macramé an attaching string for your mom. The audiologist says he thinks he can put a hook on the hearing aid."

"Oh, thank you, thank you, thank you!" I said.

JOURNAL ENTRY 7-8

Jenny called and told me Mom's new glasses had arrived a few days ago. This was good news indeed!

JOURNAL ENTRY 7-9

Mom's right hand was all curled up like a claw. It hadn't been like that the last time I'd seen her. Why hadn't someone at the nursing home told me about this over the phone? She didn't have her glasses on either. I asked her where they were.

"No good," she said.

"No, Mom, not the glasses Jenny got you from the dollar store. Your prescription glasses that are both regular glasses and bifocals."

I rummaged around in the drawer of her nightstand and found them. They were out of the case and had a smear of some kind of ointment on them. I washed them off and settled them on Mom's face.

She shook her head back and forth. "What's the matter, Mom? Can't you see better with them?"

"No good," she repeated. "No good."

I took my glasses off and put hers on, but that told me nothing. I really had no idea what her prescription should be. I called Jenny and gave her the news.

Poor Jenny. She had worked so hard to get those new glasses for Mom, following up with phone call after phone call. "I don't know what to do anymore!" she wailed.

I was stumped too. "It's just too bad her own optometrist refused to make her a new set of glasses."

"I do have her old prescription sunglasses. I found them in her purse and kept them."

"You do?" This was great news. "Maybe we can find someone who will take a reading off her prescription sunglasses and make regular glasses for her. Maybe the hospice coordinator can do something about this." I was filled with hope. Jenny wasn't as optimistic as I was.

JOURNAL ENTRY 7-10

Mom's prescription sunglasses from before her stroke arrived in the mail. I called the optometrist's name printed on the glasses case. He was the same optometrist who had told Jenny in June that he wouldn't make Mom new glasses without an in-office eye exam. I explained the situation—Mom was in a nursing home, had lost her glasses, and had to have new glasses made. I told him I doubted how useful her last eye exam had been because she hadn't been wearing her hearing aids and no family member had been there to help her communicate.

When I finished, the optometrist asked, "What is her name?"

When I told him, he looked up Mom on his computer. "I can make her a new pair of glasses."

"You can?" I was thrilled beyond belief.

"You'll need to bring in the money for payment first."

"How do I get to your office? How late are you open today?"

I arrived at the optometrist's office in less than an hour, paid cash, received the receipt, and raced back to the nursing home to tell Mom the good news—she would have a pair of *good* glasses in one week.

REPORTS FROM OTHERS

We were not alone in finding it difficult to get the nursing home to keep track of our mom's hearing aids. I wish I could report that someone I knew of had successfully managed to keep their loved one's glasses and hearing aids during the entire tenure of their nursing-home stay. Everyone I asked, even those who were otherwise satisfied with their nursing-home experience, reported that losing these items was a problem.

The website https://www.agingcare.com/ provides a forum for people to post about their own experiences. In 2015, one woman reported: "I have also had this same problem with a mother-in-law who has been in a nursing home for a year ($9,000 per month). She had spent $4,000 on a pair of hearing aids before going into the nursing home. They lost one shortly after she was in there, but she could still hear with the other one. They started locking it in a nurses cart at night so it would not get lost. Well guess what? They now lost the second one. She cannot hear at all without it. All they have offered is a stupid amplifier box that she will not use."

Samantha said the staff lost her husband's glasses on day one, and they were never found again.

Andrea, now an activities director but formerly a CNA, said, "The CNA course focuses more on the hands-on physical handling of people and incontinence. One of the biggest things you will find at any nursing home is loss of the hearing aids and dentures. It is a Bermuda Triangle or secret vortex of where these things go. You have so many different people these things pass through, and you have carelessness. Plus, young people don't realize how expensive those hearing aids are and how much people depend on them. When you don't have anything yourself that you need to depend on to see or hear, it isn't in your frame of reference. I know there isn't a lot of attention given to the hearing aids."

Claire Johnson said the nursing home refused to take any responsibility for her mother's hearing aids. They told her keeping track of the hearing aids was Claire's responsibility, not theirs.

FOR THE RECORD

Over 70 percent of nursing-home residents have hearing loss, but only 10 percent had their hearing examined in the previous year. In a study of 279 nursing-home residents, only thirty of them had had a hearing-loss screening on premises in the past year.[25] For those residents who already *do* have hearing aids, losing them is a continuous issue. Like so many other things in our United States, responsibility for replacement of hearing aids is dependent on the laws of the state which the nursing home exists.

The American Optometric Association's manual, *Optometric Care of Nursing Home Residents,* states that only 12.5 percent of nursing homes in the United States provide in-house eye care. A 1997 study showed that 30 percent of all nursing-home residents who wore glasses had difficulty seeing even with their glasses on. This would indicate an unfilled need for residents to see an eye care professional.[26]

Residents in nursing homes have the same need for ongoing monitoring of their eye health as do any other seniors. Cataracts, glaucoma, macular degeneration, and diabetes-related eye diseases all become an increasing concern in aging. Eye exams in a nursing home will likely be done with handheld instruments and lenses instead of the equipment used in an office. Depending on the patient's cognitive and physical abilities, the eye care professional may need to depend on nursing-home staff or a resident's family members to fill in certain information. It is important that an effort be made for nursing-home residents to have vision testing done.[27]

According to the National Consumer Voice, "Under the Nursing Home Reform Act of 1987, residents have the right to retain possession of their personal belongings and are entitled to a safe environment free of theft and loss." Dentures, eyeglasses, and hearing aids are included in this umbrella protection of personal belongings. Nursing homes are responsible for establishing policies to keep these items safe and to maintain an inventory list of them.[28]

TIPS

- Do not attribute hearing loss to the inevitable process of aging. Make an appointment with an audiologist for your loved one to have their hearing tested. There is a good chance the hearing loss can be remedied with the right hearing aids.
- Ask up-front about the nursing home's policies and protocols for hearing aids and glasses so there are no surprises down the road.
- Familiarize yourself with the rights of nursing-home residents in your specific state.
- Be sure to tell staff in the initial plan of care meeting—and all subsequent quarterly reviews—that your loved one wears a hearing aid.
- Have the manufacturer, model number, and serial numbers of the hearing aid written down in your records. When your loved one is admitted, ask the nursing home to sign a statement that the patient entered the facility in possession of that hearing aid.
- Use a permanent marker to write the resident's initials on the hearing aid. Try painting the hearing aid with a bright color (such as nail polish) so they are easier to spot.
- Report loss of hearing aids or glasses to your nursing-home ombudsman. Write a letter to the nursing home requesting replacement and include a date for a requested reply. If left without a response from the nursing home, you may even report this loss or theft to the police.

- Store hearing aids in a plastic case. Do not just wrap them in a tissue and put them in a drawer! They can easily wind up in the trash this way.
- Use a cord and clip system, such as the Earstay, which connects to the hearing aids on one end and clips to the resident's clothing on the other. This can keep hearing aids from hitting the floor—and possibly getting stepped on—if they fall out.[29]
- Clean the hearing aids with a soft toothbrush to remove debris when you visit.[30] Ideally, nursing-home staff would handle each resident's hearing-aid needs by cleaning them and making sure they are being used. Unfortunately, lack of time, lack of adequate staffing, and lack of training means that hearing aids are often a low priority.

CHAPTER 8
Hospice

The first person I saw when I walked into the nursing home was Heather. She had worked there for years and knew "how to get things done" better than anyone else. Heather asked me about my birthday cheesecake, something everyone knew about. My mother had talked a lot about her grand plan for my birthday. After discussing the cake, I shared with Heather my concern about Mom's condition. Heather looked down at the floor and then back at me. "Have you considered putting your mom in hospice?" she gently asked.

"Hospice?" I was startled by the suggestion. "But, but she's *here*." I had thought the nursing home itself was the final destination, the end of the line. Was there yet another stop on this one-way trip to death?

"You can be on hospice and still be here in the nursing home," Heather explained.

I hurried down the hall to Mom's room. She was curled up on her bed with a cannula pulled out of her nose while the oxygen machine rhythmically pumped away without benefiting my mom in the least.

As I reinserted the cannula into Mom's nostrils, her floor nurse came into the room and asked, "Ruth, have you considered putting your mom in hospice?"

I gulped. Part of my mind raced to remind me that death is what we had been expecting, and it was the only possible end to this story we were living through. I remembered, too, that my mother was not afraid of death. Still, this unsettled me. I replied, "No, no I hadn't. I had no idea it could be a choice."

The nurse outlined the benefits of placing Mom on hospice—Mom would have a hospice aide two hours a day, five days a week, to do anything for Mom that she wanted. An aide may read to her, put moisturizer on her skin, rub her feet, brush her hair, and help her get dressed. The benefits sounded fabulous. But I was still reeling from the word *hospice*.

Mom barely touched her lunch; she was not even interested in yogurt or the pudding I tried to spoon-feed her. She fell asleep before two o'clock, and I left to get my own lunch.

The director of nursing stopped me as I walked past her door. "Have you thought about putting your mom in hospice?" she asked. The director of nursing was a lovely woman I had spoken to a few times.

"Do you know how much it costs?" I asked. I was sure something so wonderful would cost a lot of money.

"I don't know," she answered. "You'll have to ask the social worker."

When I came back from lunch, I stopped by the social worker's office to ask her about hospice. She told me it wouldn't cost us anything and gave me brochures for two of the three hospices that worked with the nursing home; she couldn't find a brochure for the other one. I called Jenny and told her of this latest development. She was as skeptical as I was that hospice would be free.

That evening, Alberta, the night supervisor, sought me out. "I've been in this business a very long time." I had no trouble believing her. Her face was a mass of wrinkles, and she spoke with the gravelly voice of a decades-long nicotine addiction. "You get a sense for when someone is at the end of the line. I'd say your mom doesn't have very long to go."

She should have known I'd follow up with "How long do you think she has?"

Alberta was vague. "It's hard to say exactly. A few weeks maybe."

Mom was coughing a lot. The mucus coming out of her mouth was long, stringy, and sticky. It was very difficult to wipe off her face and hands. I wanted to reach down into her throat, to wherever this mucus mess came from, and yank it out by the roots. Of course, this was impossible. Her eyelashes and nostrils were caked with stuff that looked like mucus, too, so I kept washing her nose with a wet paper towel to dislodge the mucus. I almost expected to see the gunk oozing out of her ears. She didn't talk at all. I told her I would be leaving tomorrow, and she nodded her head to show she understood.

She didn't want any supper and fell asleep before they took away the food trays. I went to a restaurant with an internet connection and researched the hospice care providers on the internet. Then I called Jenny. "If it is really free," I began, "and I do find it hard to believe that it would really be free, I think we should do this for Mom."

Jenny agreed. "At least it will be one more person to pay attention to her when we aren't there."

JOURNAL ENTRY 8-2

I would return to Wisconsin later that day, and I wanted to get the ball rolling on hospice, so I went to the nursing home at 8:30 a.m. I went straight to Mindy's office. I told her Jenny and I wanted Mom to enter hospice. The social worker called hospice, and hospice called Jenny for her approval, since Jenny is Mom's health care power of attorney (POA).

The hospice nurse arrived at the nursing home and evaluated my mother right away. After, she called Jenny and set her mind at ease about payment; it would be free to us, covered by the fee we paid to the nursing home. This was incomprehensible to Jenny and me, but we were willing to give it a try.

JOURNAL ENTRY 8-3

Mom officially went into hospice today. I could hardly believe this had happened so quickly. I'd grown accustomed to a world where things happened very slowly, if at all. But, boy howdy, she was enrolled in hospice the day after our first call!

Hospice revised her drugs and took her off blood pressure medication, but it kept her on risperidone and added lorazepam. They also added morphine and a prescription for respiratory therapy. She had only been getting a medicine for her breathing that was "fast acting," but now she was also prescribed one that was long-lasting. And, as if this weren't enough, they also gave her a new air bed.

Jenny drove down from her home in northern New York and arrived in the evening. She was appalled to see Mom's poor condition.

"Should I jump on an airplane and come right back?" I queried. "Is she dying right this minute?"

"I don't know. I'll see if I can find out tomorrow."

JOURNAL ENTRY 8-4

I talked to Jenny on the phone today. She said Mom was doing better. She thought the medication changes hospice made have had a very positive impact. That horrible, sticky mucus was gone, and her breathing had improved. The hospice caregivers had been quick to tell

Jenny, though, that many hospice patients get a bounce for a week or two from going onto hospice. They cautioned her not to interpret this as Mom genuinely getting better.

We appreciated the information and were grateful for the things hospice had done. Still, we were both indignant.

We asked each other, "Why didn't her regular doctor, that idiot Dr. Adams, think to give her these different medicines?" Benign indifference or incompetence? The nursing-home staff only cared whether she was endangering her own or someone else's life. Dr. Adams needed a *specific* question before he would respond to us. Maybe if I had *asked* for these specific medications, he would have written the prescriptions. But how was I to have known that such a medication existed? Darn it all! Shouldn't he, or the nursing-home staff, have suggested all these changes on their own? Surely, these weren't secrets known only to hospice!

I tried to just be happy knowing my mom was doing better and was more comfortable. But I was more *angry* than happy.

JOURNAL ENTRY 8-5

I was absolutely stunned by the improvement in Mom's health since I had seen her just three weeks ago. She still wasn't a Chatty Cathy, but she was able to answer my questions in one or two words. I didn't hear the rattle and wheeze in her lungs as she breathed. Her mood was brighter, and she smiled when I walked into the room. I didn't care if it was the drugs that made her sweeter; I liked her this way. Actually, I loved her this way. I was smitten with my tiny, fragile mother.

"I love you, Mom," I said over and over again.

"You pity me."

I was taken aback. "Yes, Mom, I do pity you. *Of course* I pity you. You are very weak, you can't move by yourself. But," I tried to swallow past the huge lump in my throat, "I love you. Plain and simple. Not because I pity you. Just because I *do*."

She didn't say anything to that, and I sat there and held her hand until she fell asleep. Then I kept on holding it for a while longer.

JOURNAL ENTRY 8-6

I returned home to Wisconsin a few days ago. Today, I talked to Mom's hospice nurse on the phone, and she said Mom's lungs sounded clear. I told her I had found an apartment to sublet for the summer. I also asked her to tell Mom I would be there to see her next Wednesday.

Because she was with Mom right then, she put my mother on the cell phone, but it was a wretched conversation. My mom tried to talk to me, but she didn't make much sense. She would begin strong with a word or two, such as "I am," but then would trail off into silence or gibberish. It seemed she couldn't hold a thought long enough to express it.

JOURNAL ENTRY 8-7

I had several things to accomplish today. I wanted to be at the nursing home as close to eight o'clock in the morning as possible to meet Mom's new hospice aide— her third since she had been on hospice—and get the aide started off on the right foot. I wanted to show her where we kept Mom's glasses, toothbrush, hairbrush, and hearing aids. This was almost laughable because my mother had precious little storage space in the nursing home. It wasn't as if her hair brush was kept in the bedroom, the toothbrush in the bathroom, and her glasses on the mantel over the fireplace! She had only two pieces of furniture—a bookcase and a night stand. *All* of the above-mentioned items were kept in her nightstand, which had only one drawer.

Still, I wanted to have a positive attitude toward Mom's new hospice aide. I wanted to give her every possible way to succeed, so I would be there. I would show her what Mom's dark brown eyeglass case, blue toothbrush case, and bright purple, circular, metal hearing aid case all looked like.

I arrived at the nursing home at 8:15 a.m. My mom's hospice aide was supposed to be there from 8 a.m. to 10 a.m., but there was no aide. My mom looked alert. I asked her if she slept well, and she said she had even after sleeping so much during the day yesterday. This was a blessing.

I reminded Mom that she was getting her hair washed today. She nodded her head in agreement. At about eight thirty, Mom's regular nursing-home aide, Mary, came in. I asked her if she had seen Mom's new hospice aide, Woo Su.

Mary brought Woo Su into the room at 8:40 a.m. Woo Su's overall demeanor could only be described as sullen. I tried to communicate friendliness and warmth toward her as I showed her where Mom's toothbrush, hairbrush, eyeglasses, and hearing aids were kept. I said brightly, "I understand you are going to be here from eight to ten each morning."

"I have four other people I also take care of during that time period. Your mother is my fifth."

So much for the dedicated two hours of aide time from hospice!

After lunch, I pulled out three boxes of kid's flashcards with colors, shapes, numbers, and animals on them. I asked Mom to name the animals. I told myself I didn't care if she got things wrong. My goal was only to make her *talk*.

"Kangaroo, monkey, turtle." She named them without a hitch. Strangely, though, she said piano instead of skunk.

"Mom, that's not a piano. That's a *skunk*."

She studied it intently, hunching her shoulders to more closely inspect the card. I pointed at the skunk again. "Mom, what is that?"

"Porcupine," she announced.

I reminded myself of my goal and flipped to the next card. I wondered, though, about the brain chemistry that had her identify nine out of ten animals correctly, but then told her to call a skunk a piano—presumably due to its color scheme. Finally, her brain had cued her to identify the skunk as a porcupine.

JOURNAL ENTRY 8-8

Mom seemed to enjoy our work with the flashcards. But when I ventured into real-world topics, things did not go easily.

Our typical exchanges went something like this:

"Mom, are you cold?"

No answer.

"Mom, are you cold?"

I'd wait again for an answer that didn't come.

I'd ask again, more loudly this time, "Mom, are you cold?"

Silence.

Then, "Mom, can you hear me?"

"Yeth."

"Well, if you can hear me, why don't you answer me?" I was exasperated. She had her hearing aids *in*. Why were we still having these communication problems?

"No."

"No what?" My mind had been running around in circles, trying to figure out why she wasn't talking to me. Obviously, she *could* make sounds, so why wouldn't she *do* it?

"Not cold."

"Well, Mom, why couldn't you answer me before when I first asked you?" My voice betrayed my exasperation.

"I was thinking."

Oh my God, it had taken her that long to figure out if she was hot or cold and then answer such a simple question. What chance did she have of ever making her needs known to the staff, half of whom barely spoke English and all of whom were always in a rush?

JOURNAL ENTRY 8-9

Some woman came in and asked me if this was Mom's room. She wore a name tag around her neck, but as was far, far too frequent to be a coincidence, her name tag was flipped backward, unreadable.

I answered that it was Mom's room and asked who *she* was. She told me she was the substitute social worker from hospice. In the course of the conversation, I discovered she knew absolutely nothing about my mother.

She didn't know Mom's ninety-day review for hospice status was due that week, didn't know Mom's diagnosis, and didn't know who Mom's daily hospice aide was. She said the hospice staff always did patient reviews on Thursdays, but she didn't know if Mom was scheduled for this week or next week. She asked if I wanted her to call and tell me when Mom's review was scheduled.

I said yes.

Hospice did a fabulous job with Mom the first week she was with them. I never met her first aide, who quit after only one week. I didn't meet the second aide either. I'm not sure how long she stayed. Laura, the main hospice nurse, communicated with either Jenny or me fairly regularly during May and June, and we felt reassured; at least another pair of eyes were watching out for Mom. But then, in early July, the hospice organization apparently lost several staff members and Laura was moved to another facility.

After that, Mom had a series of substitute nurses. It was difficult for Jenny and me to navigate the borders of hospice and nursing-home jurisdictions. If I told hospice something first, I could sense the nursing-home staff had their noses out of joint. If I asked the nursing-home staff for something, their knee-jerk reaction was to tell me it wasn't their job because Mom was on hospice. My little mom and I were in limbo.

Mom was much better than she had been yesterday. Her mouth no longer drooped, her eyes were clear, and she drooled only a little. I found her in the dining room for lunch when I arrived. The first thing she did was ask me for a banana.

I said, "Don't you remember? I left them in your room last night."

She said she remembered, but they hadn't been there in the morning.

I looked, and sure enough, the bananas were missing. Mom asked for a banana again after a few minutes, so I called Jenny and asked her to bring a banana to the nursing home.

Mom's hospice nurse called me on the phone right after lunch. She informed me there was a note from the social worker, asking about Mom's review. The review had been that morning, and Mom had been approved to continue on hospice for another sixty days. I described to her what happened to Mom the day before and asked if she thought it had been a TIA. She said it sounded like it to her. I also asked her if Mom would continue to have small strokes and recover from them indefinitely until she had a large stroke and died. She answered that Mom was on a plateau, and that each TIA was taking a small step downward. Each TIA would erode part of her function, and although she would recover a little after each TIA, she would never fully return to where she was before the last one.

You would think I would have known this stuff by now. I thought I would have too! I wanted to join a support group for stroke patients and their families back home in Wisconsin. Unfortunately, the group nearest to me was a three-hour drive each way. The information I found on the internet was all couched in language of "each patient is unique" and "it is impossible to predict." I'd bought a book, but it had been full of medical jargon I couldn't relate to my mom.

So I was thrilled to have this information from the hospice nurse. It was the most information anyone had given me about the big picture of these strokes and TIAs, and I was grateful to get it. That evening, I rolled Mom into the lobby after dinner. I had been wondering if Mom knew, on some level, that something had been changing with her brain chemistry, but she just wasn't able to articulate questions about it. I thought she would be relieved if I brought it up and tried to explain it to her. As we sat together, I broached the topic as best as I could. "Mom, I think you had a small stroke yesterday."

She looked at me in surprise. "What makes you say that?"

I told her about her mouth slanting downward, the drool, the glazed look in her eyes, and her need for sleep.

She became very angry with me and said, "Why would you say such a terrible thing? Don't ever say such a thing again!"

"Fine, Mom. I won't say anything about it ever again." And I wouldn't. My goal was to make her as comfortable and happy as I could. If she wasn't curious about her own mental and physical state, then far be it from me to impose that knowledge on her.

JOURNAL ENTRY 8-10

What a day. I had arrived early at the nursing home, at 8:15 a.m., because Laura, Mom's original lead hospice nurse, said she would be there in the morning to look at Mom. She said she would be getting there at 7:30 a.m., would look at Mom first, and then would spend most of the morning at the nursing home.

When I walked in, Laura was examining Mom's roommate, who used the same hospice service. Mom was still in bed with no glasses and no hearing aids. I busied myself by putting those on her because if the nurse planned to ask Mom questions, it would be helpful if Mom could hear her! By 8:30 a.m., Laura had finished with the roommate. She said she needed to tell another nurse something and would be right back.

Mom's regular nursing-home nurse popped her head in to ask that we no longer leave bananas for Mom as they were drawing gnats. She said I could leave them in the kitchen refrigerator instead. I wasn't surprised by the request, but the nursing home hadn't had bananas in the kitchen for several days, which was why we had been bringing our own. I readily agreed to comply.

At 9:15 a.m., Laura still hadn't come back. When I checked the nurses' station, I saw Laura sitting there by herself. I said I would be leaving to go exercise, but I wanted her to know about a troublesome area on the back of Mom's head. I asked if Laura would please look at it. I was very nice about it and said she could give me a call when she got a chance. Laura bustled down the hall with me, muttering something about how sorry she was to have taken so long, but there had been some emergencies.

Laura looked at the mark on my mom's scalp and said she had never seen anything like it. I had shown the spot to the substitute hospice nurse last week, but apparently, she had not conveyed the information to Laura. Laura seemed genuinely surprised and perplexed by what she was seeing. She said she would have to ask the medical director about it and get back to me.

I explained I knew that because Mom was on hospice, we wouldn't be treating any skin cancer, if that was what it was. I did ask if there was something we could or should do in addition to applying a topical antibiotic ointment.

While looking at Mom's head, the hospice nurse casually mentioned that when Mom entered hospice, she had been in such bad shape, she would have died in two or three days had she not gone on hospice. Her lips were already blue.

Had I known this? Had anyone ever told me this information? I had to believe I would have acted on it and returned to the nursing home immediately if I had known!

I worked out at Curves, then showered at my apartment. When I returned to the nursing home, Mom was at her usual table for lunch with her tuna salad and mashed potatoes. *Finally, thank God,* I thought, *the correct lunch.* I'd more than once requested they serve Mom egg salad and tuna salad on alternating days as she wouldn't eat anything but mashed potatoes from their regular pureed menu. I worried she wasn't getting any protein in her limited diet of mashed potatoes and pudding.

JOURNAL ENTRY 8-11

Mom said to me, "Tomorrow, I want you to bring my walking shoes."

I was flabbergasted. "Your walking shoes? Your walking shoes have always been here. Why do you want them?"

"I am going to start walking again," she announced.

"What makes you think that?"

"I'm going to try anyway. I'm going to ask Tom—the physical therapist—if he will help me walk."

"Tomorrow is Sunday, so you'll have to wait until Monday." I shook my head, thinking she would never walk again. She hadn't placed any weight on her feet in four months. It was madness for her to think she would walk again. But if she wanted to try, and Tom was willing, I saw no harm in it.

JOURNAL ENTRY 8-12

We had a lovely time together today. Mom's roommate, Mabel, was a sweet old lady who was dying of cancer. Like the vast majority of Americans, she also loved to have the television on whenever she was in her room.

Atypically, I was raised without television for most of my childhood, partially because we were too poor to afford one, but also because my mother was opposed to television on principle. Time spent watching television was time that could be better spent reading or working. For the same reasons, I still dislike television, but if one is on in the same room with me, it is a siren I cannot ignore. Added to this was the fact that I had to speak loudly, even when Mom wore her hearing aids, so I almost gave up any attempts to converse with Mom when Mabel was in the room.

I had tried turning off the TV set when Mabel dozed off. But as we all know, turning off a television is the quickest way to wake up a sleeping person. It was like that with Mabel too. As often as possible, I took my mom outside or to the lobby. That way, we at least had a chance to converse.

Today, Mabel's family had taken her out to a restaurant for lunch, so Mom and I had the room all to ourselves. I sang to her for about two hours, checking from time to time with the daughter visiting across the hall. I wanted to be sure my singing wasn't disturbing her.

This constant communal living was one of the things I found hardest about nursing-home residence. about nursing-home residence. I often wheeled her about to the few spots a person may get a little privacy: the bench out front, the bench on the side, the courtyard, or the dining room when no one was there—which hardly ever happened as there were frequent bingo games, church groups, ice cream socials, and more. But when Mom was in bed, I had no choice but to share the room with Mabel … and her television.

Anyway, we'd had a lovely afternoon of singing. I sang the old hymns Mom loved so much: "The Old Rugged Cross," "Great Is Thy Faithfulness," "Shall We Gather at the River," and "Let the Lower Lights Be Burning." I then branched out into other songs. I sang Catholic songs in Latin: "Confitemini Domino," "Jubilate Deo," and "Magnificat." I sang one of my favorites in Spanish: "Nada Te Turbe," reminding Mom not to let anything trouble her. God alone was enough. She seemed a little impressed I could sing in a foreign language. I couldn't resist trying to show off, so I sang more songs in foreign languages for her.

JOURNAL ENTRY 8-13

If I hadn't been there to see it myself, I don't know if I would have believed it. Tom pulled Mom up onto her feet, grabbing her around the waistband of her slacks and pulling her upright. He balanced her weight on her own feet while he put her hands on the walker. Then, with me following close behind with the wheelchair, Tom and she walked down the hallway. Tom held some of her weight by pulling up on her pants, but she was moving one foot after another. She took five steps. I know because Tom counted and I saw them. She had a strong pull to the left, but she'd had that ever since the big stroke. I was truly thrilled that she was able to move so much, considering she hadn't had therapy for four months.

"Tom, thank you so much," I said with gratitude. "I wasn't sure if her feet would have pronated by now or whether they would work at all."

"Yes, people often surprise me with what they can do," Tom responded graciously. "I'll see what she's up to tomorrow."

Immediately after her walk, I took Mom to her room. "Mom, I am so proud of you!" I enthused. "You walked again. I never thought you would, but you did it, Mom. You walked again!" I could tell she was pleased with herself as well, but it goes against her religious beliefs to show pride in her own accomplishments. As a child, I had often heard, "Pride goeth before a fall."

I asked an aide to put her in bed for her nap and went to see *No Reservations,* a lovely movie starring Catherine Zeta-Jones.

On my way back from the movies, I stopped by the store to buy more bananas to satisfy Mom's insatiable banana appetite. When I walked into her room, she was in her wheelchair with her hair unbrushed (of course), but when she spotted the bananas, she was all business. "Give me that banana *now*!" she demanded. Her voice was still fragile, and the only word she actually managed was "banana," but her intent was clear! *Wow, one day of physical therapy, and she was as hungry as a horse!*

JOURNAL ENTRY 8-14

Mom was in her wheelchair already when I arrived at 11 a.m. Her glasses were on, and her hearing aids were in. She was looking down the hall, which was unusual for her. "Mom, are you looking for something?"

"Tom," was all she could manage.

"Oh," I said knowingly. "You don't want to miss Tom?"

"Yeth." She nodded.

"Well, let's go look for him, okay? We'll ask him what time he thinks he will get to you today." I pushed her down the hallway.

Tom said he was free at the moment and would take Mom right away. Lucky for us!

Therapy, at first, appeared to be a repeat of yesterday's routine. I expected he would try to have her take *six* steps so she could feel good about the improvement over the day before. But much to my amazement, she took *fifteen*! Not only did she take that many steps, but Tom also wasn't holding up her weight as much as he had the day before. I was flummoxed.

Afterward, I casually asked Mom why she suddenly wanted to walk again. It sounded liked she said, "Ethel."

"Ethel?" I queried disbelieving.

"Yeth," she confirmed.

A light slowly dawned. "Do you mean Ethel who is a resident here?"

"Yeth."

Egads. Ethel, Ethel, Ethel. Poor thing, she was one of only three patients in the nursing home who could still walk without a cane or a walker. She was the one who tried to help poor old Lucy the other day. But Ethel was quickly losing all her marbles. I knew this because I was here so much, the staff sometimes slipped and talked about other patients within my earshot. And, yes, it made sense. Ethel did walk past Mom's door nearly every time I sat beside her. And when Mom was in bed, Ethel would say, "What are you doing in bed? You need to get up and get moving!"

I didn't realize Mom was taking Ethel's comments so much to heart. But isn't it amazing how much of an influence one person can have on another person even if they have dementia and don't realize the impact of what they are saying? It makes you stop and think about the unintended consequences of things we say to others as well!

JOURNAL ENTRY 8-15

Tom had been off work yesterday so Mom didn't get a chance to walk. She was raring to go when I arrived today. She barely tolerated me turning on her hearing aids and brushing her hair. She wanted to go find Tom!

Unfortunately, I lost count of how many steps she took today. Tom didn't hold on to her waistband at all once she got on her feet; he just held her under one arm. She didn't veer off to the left very much. She walked, actually *walked* with a step, not a shuffle. I knew it had to have been more than fifteen steps, but I couldn't say how many. I was so surprised, I almost forgot to push the wheelchair behind her to sit down when Tom decided she'd had enough.

She had drawn a small crowd of staff members with this amazing feat. By the end of the day, however, Tom told me he wasn't allowed to do therapy with my mom again because she was on hospice. We had heard from several other sources that residents on hospice can't have therapy. He was sorry about it, and he had hoped to keep it secret, but with everyone gathered around her today, the word had quickly spread back to the administration. I would have to get permission from the director of nursing for Mom to continue therapy, and he didn't think permission was likely.

JOURNAL ENTRY 8-16

Jenny and I talked today to Joanne, the director of nursing at Pineville, about taking Mom off hospice. We told her we had heard that a patient couldn't concurrently be on hospice and receive physical therapy. She confirmed this. We asked if she thought we would be doing Mom any harm by going off hospice. She said not at all, that Mom seemed to be stable, and furthermore, a patient could go back on hospice at any time they chose as long as their condition warranted it.

Still grateful for the help hospice had provided by changing Mom's medications last May and providing a better bed for her, we emphasized we would be going off hospice for the physical therapy.

Joanne, unfortunately for us, had her own axe to grind with hospice. We soon came to understand she was unhappy with the service this particular hospice program provided. When we told Joanne we definitely wanted to take Mom off hospice, Joanne insisted she should call hospice herself.

She decided to use us as a case in point to express her own unhappiness with the hospice program. She told them we were dissatisfied with the aides provided (this was true), lack of music therapy (also true), lack of aromatherapy (definitely *not* true; we were never even told this was an option), and lack of massage (also not true).

That night, Jenny and I each got distressed calls from Laura, the hospice nurse, who asked us to call her to discuss the decision. She said there would be paperwork for us to sign to remove Mom from hospice and she would see us tomorrow.

JOURNAL ENTRY 8-17

Jenny and I arrived at Pineville together in the morning so as to present a united front to Laura. We told her we made our decision because Mom wanted physical therapy. Laura immediately said hospice would provide Mom with physical therapy if we wanted it.

We were nonplussed. "But we were told you couldn't be on hospice *and* get physical therapy at the same time!"

"That is generally true. But we can make exceptions in special cases. I've already talked to my supervisor about this, and she said to make you this offer."

Jenny and I went off to discuss. When Brenda, the floor nurse, walked by, we asked her opinion. Brenda said we should be sure that whomever hospice provided for therapy was licensed and supervised. She also implied that if Mom was injured in therapy with a therapist from hospice, there may be some delicate negotiations about who was at fault.

My mind quickly flashed back to how difficult it had been to establish who had last seen Mom's hearing aids, the hospital or the nursing home. I also thought about how quick the nursing home was to tell me that anything from weighing Mom to getting her cough medicine was something hospice was supposed to do.

But when I would ask hospice, they were adamant I ask the nursing home to do it as it was the nursing home's job. I really didn't want to go through more of that ask-your-father-ask-your-mother routine.

Jenny and I told Laura we were firm in our decision to take Mom off hospice for a reason that was true: we had been disappointed about the lack of music therapy. I told her we had chosen her specific hospice over the other two specifically for that service.

Laura replied, at first, that it was too difficult to get volunteers to do music therapy. Then she said that maybe, once school started, she could find some schoolkids who would sing to Mom after school.

I was truly surprised by this suggestion, so I asked, "But will these kids know the old-time songs? Mom likes songs such as 'Bicycle Built for Two,' 'Has Anybody Seen my Girl?,' and 'Ain't She Sweet?,' as well as the old church songs."

Laura brightened. "I know what your Mom needs—a tape player in her room. Then she can play tapes of the music she likes."

"Laura," I explained. "I bought Mom a tape player back in February. I bought her one with earphones so she wouldn't bother anyone else and would have a better chance of hearing it. The problem is that Mom cannot reach anything unless it is on her tray table that slides over her bed. But you can't keep a tape player on the tray table because when they bring in her food, they have to move it. When they give her a bath, they would have to move it. And then, unless someone puts it back on the tray table again, she can't reach it. And further, there is no electrical outlet that can be reached when it is on the tray table unless there is a long extension cord. You know what that means—a tripping hazard. No, Laura, we tried a tape player, and it didn't work."

Laura thought for a moment, then said, "I know, we can have the hospice aide turn the radio on for her while she gets her dressed in the morning and turn it off when she leaves."

Jenny and I were dumbfounded. Mom had been on hospice for four months, and the only idea they can come up with for "music therapy" was an aide playing the radio for fifteen minutes each day?

At that, Jenny asked for the paperwork and signed for Mom to be removed from hospice.

What we had most hoped for from hospice—an aide who would not only develop a personal relationship with Mom after being with her ten hours each week, but would also be additional eyes and ears to track her condition—had not materialized. This failed due to hospice staffing problems and language difficulties with the staff members they did provide. Furthermore, even with the hospice aide, Mom was still showing up in the dining hall for lunch without her hearing aids turned on and, sometimes, without her glasses. This was the most serious deficit Jenny and I noted.

JOURNAL ENTRY 8-18

When I arrived this morning, my mom wasn't in her room or the dining room, so I peeked into the therapy room. I was happy to see she was working with a physical therapist who had her reaching up to take brightly colored cones from a stack and place them on the floor. The therapist was having trouble getting Mom to hear her, so I went in and checked her hearing aids. They were not turned on. Getting a nursing-home employee to turn on Mom's hearing aids was an ongoing struggle I was never going to win. But I had thought a physical therapist would be thoughtful enough to check and see if a person's hearing aids were working. Apparently not! I turned on Mom's hearing aids so she could hear the therapist. Sigh.

Afterward, I met with her physical therapists—she had more than one due to scheduling—to ask about Mom's possible outcome from therapy. They both said she had potential; she just hadn't reached yet. They were proud of how far she walked, although she did have a pronounced list, or tilt, to the left they were trying to correct. They said they would keep her for at least three weeks on therapy before putting her back on restorative therapy, where they do little.

I then went down and told Mom I had gotten her report card from therapy, and they had said she was doing really well. She was so happy. What a smile on her face! "Oh," she said. "Really? I thought I did lousy." I assured her she was doing a great job, and I was really proud of her.

JOURNAL ENTRY 8-19

Mom began major therapy, both physical therapy and occupational therapy today. Last night, she practiced talking with me. It came out mostly as incoherent gobbledygook. But the *intention* to actually communicate a complex thought was there. All summer, I'd had to coax her to utter even single syllables. Once in a while, she would spontaneously say "drink" if she wanted a drink, or "banana" if she wanted one of those. But mostly, it had been me showing her pictures in books or flashcards or asking questions in an attempt to keep her verbal at all.

Out of the blue, she said, "I want to learn to walk on my own again." She had said that a week or so ago, and that had started the process that led to leaving hospice. Apparently, she had been thinking it over and was affirming her decision.

"That would be great, Mom." I felt no need to have her dial down her dreams. If she *does* learn to walk again, that would be wonderful. There are those who will think it unseemly and a waste of society's resources for an eighty-nine-year-old woman who would never again be "productive" to learn to walk. But I was thinking each day was a gift. If those days are given at eighty-nine, they are still a gift. Who was I to spit in the eye of a benevolent God and say, "Hey, we don't want these precious moments because we know they won't be leading to full recovery. Take this away from us." On my mother's behalf, I accepted this gift for however long it would last.

FOR THE RECORD

The word "hospice" originally meant "a place of shelter." In 1974, the first hospice in the United States opened in New Haven, Connecticut. In 2012, there were more than 5,500 hospice programs in the United States Although many Americans use hospice care during their final days, two-thirds of them receive these services in their own home. About 1.6 million patients enter hospices each year with Medicare covering the costs for 84 percent; 0.6 percent are self-pay, and the remainder are covered by Medicaid.[31]

Hospice is not always an actual, physical place dedicated to hospice services. Hospice services can be provided to patients in nursing homes, hospitals, or in their own homes. They provide services, including bereavement counseling, to the family as well as the patient.

Despite the prevalence of hospices today, there are still some misconceptions about what it means to be in hospice. Everyone should know that:

a) Hospice is for those people with limited life expectancies, but it does not mean you have given up on living. In fact "research shows that hospice recipients live longer, on average, than those receiving standard care. One 2010 study of lung cancer patients found that they survived nearly three months longer."[32]

b) Hospice does not drug people to hasten their death. Drugs are used for pain management only.

c) Hospice is not a permanent commitment. You can choose to withdraw at any time for any reason. You can return to hospice later if you so choose.

TIPS

- Choose a hospice that is Medicare certified if you plan to have Medicare pay for a hospice stay. A *Huffington Post* survey in 2014 revealed that over 750 hospices in the United States had not had an inspection in over six years. Those uninspected hospices were not Medicare certified as regular inspections are required by Medicare.[33]

- Look for a hospice's accreditation. Accreditation is not required by Medicare for payment, but the National Hospice and Palliative Care Organization and the Community Health Accreditation Partner both offer additional accreditation to show that a facility meets certain standards of excellence. Also, check to see if the medical director of the hospice is board certified in palliative medicine.

- Ask about the caseload of their hospice nurses or nurse practitioners. Ideally, they should not be expected to manage a caseload of more than twelve patients.

- Ask probing questions about how often and by whom special services, such as massage or music therapy, will be provided.

CHAPTER 9
Grooming

I arrived at the nursing home at 11:30 a.m. Mom was already in the dining room, seated at the table for people who need help with eating. Poor little thing looked like a ragamuffin. Her hair wasn't brushed, she had no glasses on, and her hearing aids weren't in. She was slumped to one side and drooling.

I swooped in and wheeled her away from the table and back to her room, where I brushed her hair, put on her glasses, and put in her hearing aids. "There, Mom," I said cheerily, "Don't you feel better now?"

"Yeth." She agreed, and I wheeled her back to the regular dining room that featured wall-to-wall carpet and a piano.

Honestly, I thought, *I don't know what is wrong with those aides that they didn't brush her hair and put in her hearing aids. Maybe they didn't know about the new glasses. That I could overlook, but the hair and hearing aids—that just wasn't right!*

JOURNAL ENTRY 9-2

I wanted to make sure Mom had her hair washed and styled at the beauty parlor located on the premises of the nursing home. Phyllis, the hairdresser who came into the nursing home, did a good job of fixing the residents' hair, but last week, Mom had refused to have her hair shampooed. I'd spoken with her about this more than once in the past few days, and she was on board with getting her hair washed this week.

It had been three weeks without a shampoo, and her hair was looking dirty and gross. She hadn't wanted to get it done because "it didn't last"—a day after her last wash and style, I had plonked a sun hat on top of her head, and it irked her that I had ruined her hair. I explained that even if the styling didn't last, then at least her hair would be clean. Besides, we'd already paid for it.

JOURNAL ENTRY 9-3

Mom's floor nurse found me today and explained that if we wanted Mom to be seen by a dentist, we would have to make a specific request. I had thought dental care was regularly provided at the nursing home. Apparently, dental cleanings were *not* part of services provided there by the visiting dentist. According to the floor nurse, a dentist came every two weeks (who knew?) and would do extractions, but he didn't normally clean teeth. For that service, we would have to pay $140 out of pocket. I said I would be happy to pay that. Then she mentioned something about needing to send a fax, but she also said she would follow up on it. I decided I'd wait a few days and then track her down again if she didn't come and find me.

I truly did not understand this. At least half the people in this nursing home had been residents for more than two years. Some had been here for over ten years. Did this mean they didn't get their teeth cleaned? No wonder many residents' teeth looked so bad. Dental care was something I had been wondering about for some time. Mom had always gone every six months for a dental cleaning, but she hadn't had one now for over a year. Jenny and I had been relieved when we saw the box to check for dental care in the admitting paperwork. Jenny had asked Mindy, the social worker at the nursing home, about teeth cleaning in February, the last time Mom had come back from the hospital. Mindy had said she would take care of it. Yeah, right! At that time, our energies with the nursing home had been taken up with getting her new glasses and hearing aids.

And I wondered again what would happen to me if I were someday a nursing-home resident. I have no children to fight these battles for me. No one who would think, *Hmmmm, it has been over a year since she has seen a dentist, so whom do I ask to make this happen?* Obviously, arrangement for eyeglasses, hearing aids, and dental checkups are not automatically handled in a nursing home!

JOURNAL ENTRY 9-4

This morning, I stopped by to see Mom early—around nine o'clock—to let her know I had not forgotten her and would be back to have lunch with her. At that time, she was still lying in bed in her nightgown, with no glasses or hearing aids, of course. But when she saw me, her face opened into a smile, and I was glad I had come. Shortly after my arrival, her aide showed up to get Mom dressed and ready for the day. I ran into her floor nurse and she said, "It is on my list of things to do today to contact the dentist and get that paperwork for you to sign."

I assured her I had my checkbook with me and would write a check on the spot; she had only to tell me who to make it out to. She said she would get back to me.

The dental situation made me wonder, *What is the value of a life like my mother's?* She consumed a tremendous amount of energy from those who were able-bodied. The nursing-home staff cooked her food and washed her dishes. Jenny and I spent at least four hours of our time visiting her each day. We made my mother pureed chicken and ham salads to tempt her palate. Someone from Mom's church visited her at least twice a week. An entire staff kept the nursing-home building clean and safe. It would be interesting to divide all these hours by the number of patients and see how many person-hours of effort it took to keep each patient going. I guessed it was my training in economics that inclined me to consider a cost-benefit analysis.

Objectively, one may say my mother gave very little back to anyone. She was querulous with the staff and other patients. She did not want to participate in any group activities. Her minister had wanted her to attend a special service the following month at the church to honor its senior citizens, and my mother adamantly refused this request. This perplexed me as she was obviously loved by her church community. I asked her why, and she explained she didn't want anyone to see her the way she was. At eighty-nine, she was still vain about her appearance!

JOURNAL ENTRY 9-5

This morning, Mom's mouth was pulled down on one side. Drool ran down her chin and soaked her blouse, and her eyes were glazed. I held her hand and put my arm around her shoulders. I could see she was having a difficult time. She managed to eat a little lunch, then fell asleep with her head dropped forward like a sunflower past its prime. It looked like a very uncomfortable position. I asked an aide to put her to bed before it was even one o'clock.

It broke my heart to see her like that. I hated to see neurological impulses beyond her control twist her face and numb her mind. I believed she was having another stroke. But since she had a do-not-hospitalize (DNH) order, there was nothing for me to do and nothing I could ask the staff to do.

After they put her in bed, I went to the store and bought a farewell card for my friend Fern, who was leaving the next day to return home to Colorado. Fern had been around for almost a year, caring for her father who had Alzheimer's and still lived at home. Now, it was time for her sister Rose to take a turn. Fern's family was wealthy enough to afford a live-in caregiver in addition to the family's help. And really, I could see how they would need to have two people on hand to keep her father safe.

When I returned to the nursing home a little after four o'clock, Mom was still sleeping. She woke up when they brought in the dinner trays, and I didn't ask them to get her up and into her wheelchair. I fed her in bed and then sang to her. Some days, she tried to sing along or at least mouthed the words. Today, she did not. The only thing she asked me for was a banana, and I didn't have any. The nursing-home kitchen had none either. Frustrated, I bought three for her at the grocery store. I left them on her bookcase so she could have one with her breakfast in the morning.

JOURNAL ENTRY 9-6

I asked Mom's floor nurse today whether she had the paperwork for me to sign for Mom's dental cleaning. She said the dentist office had called her and explained their standard practice. First, they conducted an exam for $75. Then, they did the cleaning for $140. If I didn't want the exam, I would have to sign a waiver to that effect.

"Yes, fine, I will sign the waiver. We just want her teeth cleaned." How long had it been? At least two weeks, and I was still simply trying to get the paperwork completed so Mom could get on the list to have her teeth cleaned.

JOURNAL ENTRY 9-7

The floor nurse caught me in the hall and gave me the permission slip for the dentist. Jenny, who held Mom's health care POA, would have to sign it, but at least we had it. I could only hope it would turn out to be the correct form!

JOURNAL ENTRY 9-8

This was the fifth day in a row I had walked into the nursing home at 11:30 a.m. to find my mom up, dressed, and in the dining room but still without her glasses or hearing aids. I wheeled Mom back to her room for these important items. There, I put her glasses on her face and her hearing aids into her ears. The hearing aids were so small that I was never sure if I had the little dial on the right setting for the volume. I had devised a little hearing aid routine where I stand behind her and say, "Mom, can you hear me? If you can hear me, tell me what color I am saying. The color is red—or blue, green, and so on." If she didn't say anything, I knew I needed to turn the volume up higher.

Jenny signed the permission form for the dentist. I mailed it along with a check for $140 today. Now, we just had to wait and see how long it would be before her cleaning—don't get me started on this frustrating fact; the aides did not bother to even hand her a toothbrush so she could at least *try* to brush her teeth each day.

JOURNAL ENTRY 9-9

The dentist finally came to clean Mom's teeth. What a long process it had been to get this to happen. Jenny had first requested this of the social worker at the nursing home over six months ago. But then, Mom's glasses suddenly went missing, then her hearing aids too. After that, she went on hospice, and we spent months thinking she would die soon. Finally, I thought, *Hey, no one is giving us a timetable for anything, so she might live several more years. Why should the poor thing wind up with cavities if she doesn't have to?* So I decided to pursue a dentist visit for Mom.

The nursing home had said it had a dentist who visited regularly, but here was the real scoop: the dentist told me she could do extractions, but she could not do fillings. She could "sort of" do a teeth cleaning, but even the dentist admitted it wasn't very thorough. But still, something was better than absolutely nothing. I mean, just because Mom was in a nursing home didn't mean her teeth wouldn't decay and her gums wouldn't develop problems just as they would have had she lived at home. And with the poor dental hygiene visited upon her since the big stroke, well, it was high time for her to see a dentist!

The dentist said Mom's teeth were in very good shape for a woman of her age, but she did have three cavities. I got the impression they weren't that bad yet because Mom hadn't complained about feeling any pain. Still, I had to figure out how to get the cavities taken care of.

JOURNAL ENTRY 9-10

Yesterday was a very hard day. I felt like I had not been spending enough quality time with my mom over the last few days. I had been at the nursing home, but I stayed busy with other issues, chatted with other people, and didn't spend the unstructured and undivided attention time with my mom the way she likes. To be honest, I enjoyed that time, too, so I came to the nursing home early to spend more time with her.

I got there about ten o'clock. First thing I noticed was that her bed was unplugged again, a near daily occurrence. Her bed was an air bed, and when it wasn't plugged into the wall, it lost all of its air. Mom was left lying on the solid bottom, so I plugged in her bed. I certainly knew where the outlet was by now.

I washed her glasses. I brushed her hair and set her up to brush her teeth. I had been remiss about this—the only thing I felt guilty about. I hadn't been as diligent as I should have been about toothbrushing. I had let myself assume that the aides were doing this, but I now knew I had been kidding myself.

I set her up with one cup of water to dunk her toothbrush in and another one for her to spit into. I retrieved her little, pink, kitty cat toothbrush and put a dab of toothpaste on it. I put a bib on her so she wouldn't get her shirt wet and messy. I put the toothbrush in her hand, and she set to the task. Meanwhile, I busied myself with the plants on her windowsill. I did go change the water in her cup a few times.

While this was going on, Debbie, the floor nurse, walked in and noticed the toothbrushing. She said, "Oh gosh, I know the aides aren't very good about doing that. I've been meaning to talk to them about it."

I felt very virtuous after all of this grooming. I put Mom's little, pink bonnet on her head, exchanged her sunglasses for her regular glasses, put an afghan on her knees in case she would think it was chilly, and then rolled her outdoors. It was a beautiful, perfect morning, and I felt very pleased with myself.

I asked Mom, "How did it feel to brush your teeth this morning?" During my last week there, I had decided I would make toothbrushing my last battle with the nursing home.

"If you can call it brushing your teeth! I'd rather go jump in the lake!"

I was startled by this response. "What? What do you mean? What else did you need to brush your teeth?"

"I need more water, a pitcher of water, and a basin to spit into."

"You mean to tell me that the cup isn't enough for you to spit into?" I felt quite annoyed by this ingratitude.

"No, it isn't. I need a basin."

I hadn't bothered to hope that even the modest setup I had provided for her would be replicated by the nursing-home staff. To date, it had been a struggle just to get them to put her glasses on her face and her hearing aids in her ears. Even when they managed these tasks, the glasses were invariably dirty, and the hearing aids were rarely turned on. Thus far, they hadn't managed to fish her toothbrush out of her drawer and put it in her hand. To request more than the simple setup I gave Mom this morning would be futile.

Frustrated and more than a little angry, I burst out, "You are so ungrateful!"

"I just want to die. I pray every day that I will die. That's all I want to do."

"I don't believe you want to die. You are asking for therapy. You want to walk again. These are not signs of a person who wants to die. These are signs of a person who wants to live, who wants to get better. Personally, I don't care if you do learn to walk again or not. It is up to you. But Jenny and I have had to go to a lot of work and trouble and get special permission for you to have therapy again. And if you do want to try to walk again, you are going to have to put forth a lot of effort. If you don't show improvement, they will drop you from therapy."

Then I gave her a little public service announcement about the importance of eating some protein-rich food every day. This was another item we had persistently struggled to obtain for her.

Mom's ongoing swallowing problems and aspiration risk meant she was still on pureed foods only. The nursing home did put a pureed meat product on her food tray every day. I knew it was nutritious, but it looked awful. I had never seen her, not once, stick her spoon in any of the pureed meat on her tray. But she would eat egg salad and tuna salad, so Jenny and I had gone round and round among the dining room aides, the social worker, floor nurse, speech therapist—because the speech therapist is the expert on swallowing to ensure they would serve Mom tuna salad or egg salad each day at lunchtime. They also put yogurt on her tray for supper, and I often brought in little cups of cottage cheese, both of which she had outright refused for several weeks. She would eat the egg salad only if I spooned it into her mouth, and she grudgingly ate a few spoons of tuna if I insisted.

I had already explained more than once the importance of protein foods in her diet. I had also tried, unsuccessfully, to help her memorize the four protein foods available at the nursing home I thought she would eat: tuna, eggs, cheese, and yogurt. She wouldn't listen to my dietary lecture, though, so I let it drop.

FOR THE RECORD

Dental care. It is estimated that as many as 80 percent of residents in long-term care facilities do not receive a daily toothbrushing.[34] Frank A. Scannapieco, a professor and chair of oral biology at the State University of New York at Buffalo, studied the effect of mouth bacteria on overall health. He postulated that bacteria in the mouth can often lead to pneumonia. In one study, it was found that the bacteria in the lungs of patients with pneumonia was identical to the bacteria cultured from the teeth of those same patients.[35] At least fifteen studies have shown that daily oral hygiene decreased aspiration pneumonia.[36]

Many nursing-home patients are unable to brush and floss on their own, much less meticulously, so it is advantageous for nurses or aides to perform this on a daily basis. Scannapieco stated that toothbrushing and flossing would help somewhat to remove harmful bacteria, but a dental cleaning by a dentist or hygienist is best. According to a 2019 article, only 10.3 percent of patients admitted to a nursing home received dental services from a dentist or dental hygienist.[37]

Daily oral hygiene in long-term care facilities is further complicated when residents have diabetes or swallowing precautions. Inability to sit or stand upright also make it difficult. Using suction toothbrushes and raising the head of the bed can ameliorate some of these issues. It is critical that staff wear fresh, clean gloves to provide oral care and not touch anything but the patient's mouth while those gloves are on.

Patients with cognitive impairments can present challenges for any staff person who would assist with or provide dental hygiene. A study of CNAs who had been given specific training on this found that even with training, only 16 percent felt comfortable providing these services.[38]

California standards specifically state that "nursing homes must assist residents in obtaining routine and emergency dental care. Routine care means an annual exam." Unfortunately, such dental services are not covered by Medicare and rarely by Medicaid. Yet, under federal law, nursing homes should provide both routine and emergency dental care. Something called "Incurred Medical Expense" (IME) can pay for dental care, eye glasses, and hearing aids. IME requires monthly payments, and arrangements must be made with the nursing home's administration. It is something like a loan to be repaid from the resident's monthly personal allowance.[39]

Cutting nails. It had long frustrated me that no one on staff would cut or file my mother's fingernails. They were also filthy if neither Jenny nor I had been there in more than a week. When we had asked about fingernail cutting, we were told by the CNAs that they were not permitted to do anything with nails. I had assumed this was a governmental regulation, but Bridget Malkin's article in *Nursing Times* clarified that the "rule" against nurses cutting fingernails or toenails is a myth.[40]

A training manual for CNAs includes detailed information on how to keep nails clean and trimmed. This manual gives justifications for CNAs providing this service:

1. An unconscious patient with long nails can scratch her own skin, leading to infection.
2. Nail beds can harbor microorganisms that can cause infection.
3. Fungal growth in the nail bed can lead to permanent damage to the nail or infection and needs to be reported to the nurse.

These detailed instructions for nail care include the caveat that CNAs should not be cutting the nails of patients who take anticoagulation drugs or are diabetic.

My mother was not diabetic nor was she taking anticoagulation drugs. The nursing home probably established the rule to shorten time spent in direct patient care. Or, perhaps, they exercised an overabundance of caution to make sure an aide didn't accidently cut the nails of anyone who shouldn't have had their nails cut. But I always wondered, *Who cuts the fingernails of people who don't have children or friends to come in and see to their nails?*

TIPS

- Visitors to residents in health-care facilities should look at the nails of the resident. If you feel squeamish about doing this, *Nursing Times* suggests you remind yourself of the effect of uncut fingernails on infection rates.
- Frank A. Scannapieco said toothbrushing and flossing will improve dental health, but for them to be effective, they must be done several times each day. Other methods, including rinses of chlorhexidine and betadine and toothbrushing by staff, will also improve dental hygiene. However, nothing can take the place of a professional cleaning with sharp instruments or ultrasonic scalers.[41]
- Lack of good personal hygiene, including dental care and clipping of fingernails, is one of six red flags you should watch for when monitoring a loved one's care in a nursing home.[42]

CHAPTER 10
Paperwork

Mom's DNH order became a very important piece of paperwork to us after her transport from the nursing home to a hospital. This is what happened.

JOURNAL ENTRY 10-1

My husband, Luke, and I flew into Philadelphia, rented a car, and drove straight to the hospital. There was a neon-green sign posted on the door of Mom's room saying visitors should check in at the nurses' station first before entering because patients in this room were contagious. The sign stipulated that visitors should wear gloves, refrain from touching the patients, and wash their own hands thoroughly upon leaving.

At the nurses' station, I identified myself as my mother's daughter and asked the reason for the precautions.

"Oh, we can't tell you that. You'll have to ask her doctor."

This angered me. "Why is the sign up there then?"

"You should definitely wash your hands thoroughly when you leave her room. Don't touch her bodily fluids or anything that could have her fluids on it, like a dirty tissue."

"Does my mother still have pneumonia?"

"I can't tell you that. You'll have to ask her doctor."

"She's been here for over a week and isn't using oxygen. Do you think she will go home soon?"

"I can't tell you anything. You'll have to ask her doctor."

I went from angry to defeated in less than one minute. I had worked as both a journalist and as a lawyer, and yet I always felt like I hit an insurmountable wall with this noncommunicative hospital.

I could have become belligerent. I could have pitched a fit. I could have requested to speak with a supervisor, administrator, or state senator. But I knew, all too well, that I was at the hospital for only a few days and then only for seven or eight hours each day. If I made enemies there, the hours when I was absent could be very uncomfortable for my mother. There were dozens of little ways they could make her life miserable even without endangering her—not bringing a spoon for her yogurt, not opening her container of nectar juice, or leaving her to lie in her own wastes for an extra hour. Yes, I knew there were (and still are) many dedicated staff people working in hospitals all over the world.

I just didn't know if any of them worked where my mother was hospitalized.

I walked into my mom's room to find her shrunken and shivering form huddled under a sheet. Her hair, pure white now, was standing straight up on top of her head.

I asked her if she knew where her hairbrush, glasses, or hearing aids were. She couldn't answer me. Her eyes were open, and she had an expression on her face like that of a startled animal. She did say my name once, so I knew she was awake, but, otherwise, she didn't communicate. I searched her one drawer and looked around the floor. There was no other place to check for her personal items.

I wear glasses from the minute I wake up until I fall asleep. I would be lost and disoriented without them. I would have a headache. If I were deprived of my glasses, I know I would be very cranky. Mom had nothing to read. Her television set was on but perpetually showed the timetable for in-hospital health programs. No one had visited her to pay for her TV channels, but her eyes were often trained on the screen nonetheless. A frosted-over window permitted light and a chilly draft, but the view was a brick wall about ten feet away. She must have been bored and miserable.

"Mom, are you cold?"

She nodded her head.

"Luke," I said, "go find my mother a blanket!"

I draped my coat across her body and bent to cradle her in my arms. I noticed she couldn't turn on her side because a black strap across her chest restrained her.

"I'm your mom's roommate," said a voice from the other side of the curtain. "They have her doped up on haloperidol because she has been giving them a hard time."

I introduced myself to Mom's roommate, Jolene. "What has she been doing?" I asked, full of dread.

"Well, she told me I was Judas Iscariot and was going to burn in hell. She said some of the nurses have hellfire shooting out of their eyes. And she has been asking for a diaper over and over again. Finally, she tried to make a diaper for herself out of the sheets, and they didn't like that one bit. That's when they restrained her hands. I don't blame her, myself."

I didn't blame her, either. I knew how long they made a patient wait to get changed.

I asked Jolene why she was in the hospital. Jolene explained she was infected with MRSA, and my mom must have been too; she reasoned they wouldn't put two patients in the same room if they weren't both infected.

Luke returned with one thin blanket—it was all he could find. We put it on my mom, but she still shivered. Luke went to ask someone for another blanket. He returned with a pile of three sheets. The aide said there were no more blankets on the floor, so we'd have to make do with these sheets. She suggested we bring in a blanket from home.

Having spent three years living in Venezuela, I was familiar with hospitals without sheets or blankets for patients. Heck, in Venezuela they didn't have medicine, blood for transfusions, or even *food* in the hospitals.

Families and friends were expected to bring all of these items to the hospital. Still, I never dreamed I'd be experiencing this in a large hospital in New Jersey.

When the supper tray arrived, I managed to coax my mother to eat some mashed potatoes and yogurt. The nurse came in while I was doing this and said, "That's good. She didn't eat any of her lunch today. I couldn't even wake her up."

"Oh." I tried to make my voice casual and kept my eyes on the floor. "Is that because she was on haloperidol?"

"Yeah, it could have been the haloperidol making her sleep."

I silently thanked Jolene for tipping me off. I knew by then that the staff would never admit anything unless I guessed at it first. "I'll be bringing her glasses and hearing aids tomorrow. Maybe some socks, a sweater, and a blanket. That should make a difference."

"Well, I'm not sure that is such a good idea. We can't keep track of glasses and hearing aids. And we definitely don't keep track of socks and sweaters. When we change her, we'll just toss them into the laundry. She'll never get them back. But a little throw blanket might be good."

JOURNAL ENTRY 10-2

We arrived bright and early at the hospital. I brought a blanket, a box of tissues, hand lotion, her hairbrush, and her glasses. The hearing aids—costing over $6,000—were too expensive to risk losing; they remained at the nursing home. That was why I knew later on that the hospital had not lost her hearing aids—I had never taken them there to begin with.

I popped her glasses on her face and brushed her hair down. She wasn't Miss America, but at least she didn't look like a troll doll any more. Her cranberry-colored throw blanket brought a little color to a room that was, otherwise, as drab as a prison cell.

She seemed a little more alert than she had been yesterday, maybe because she had her glasses on. She tried more than once to talk. She would start off by saying, "What I want to tell you is" or "What I am trying to say," then she would lose her focus and stop talking. I guessed for her in hopes of helping her complete a sentence.

I would venture, "Food. Mom, were you going to tell me something about food?"

Pause. No response.

"Pain? Mom, are you having pain somewhere?"

This would go on until I ran out of guesses. She gave no response one way or another.

I asked her roommate, Jolene, if they had given my mom haloperidol in the morning. "They said she was in such a good mood, they would try skipping the haloperidol today."

I wondered how long it took for haloperidol to pass out of the system. Was she zoned out and unable to hold a thought for more than five seconds because of the haloperidol, or had she suffered another stroke? By that point, I knew better than to ask the nursing staff any questions.

Jolene had some serious problems of her own. In one leg, her bones had broken in several places. The metal rod the doctors had originally placed in her leg had become infected, so now big, vicious-looking screws locked an external metal rod onto her leg. She said half her hip had also been removed. They had allowed this incision to drain, and so much blood dripped out of it that even though I had given her five absorbent pads from the pile on the windowsill—which she couldn't have reached on her own—she was still bleeding. Of course, the nursing staff was taking their sweet time to respond to her call button. Finally, an aide walked in, switched off the call button, and turned to leave.

"This woman is bleeding," I shouted.

The aide then went over, looked at Jolene, and said, "I'll get a nurse."

The nurse came in and examined it. "Oh, that isn't so bad," she scoffed.

So much for the theory they only pay attention to you if you are bleeding. They don't pay attention to you here even if you *are* bleeding.

Mom's minister arrived shortly after I gave up on feeding her any supper. He had been very faithful about visiting her. He tried conversing with her, and when that didn't work, he started to read from Scripture.

Mom interrupted him. "You, you, you." She struggled with the words but finally managed to sputter, "You have been telling the congregation that I am a lunatic!"

At that point, I excused myself. *If the shoe fits, Mom,* I thought. I was helpless in the face of mental illness. Didn't this have to be some form of mental illness? I knew so little about it and had no diagnosis for her. My only clue to a diagnosis was that she had been dosed with both risperidone and haloperidol for short periods since her stroke.

I thought I had been mentally prepared, ready for senility, dementia, or Alzheimer's. But this looked like a possible form of insanity. Or had her symptoms simply been induced by the haloperidol? Which had come first, the haloperidol or the hallucinations?

After the minister finished with my mother, he took me aside in the hallway. "This might not be any of my business, but I thought I would ask if your mother has an advance medical directive. I'm asking because I think they might want to put the feeding tube back in her stomach."

"Yes, she does have an advance medical directive and she specifically stated she doesn't want that again. She said it to my sister, to me, and to my husband. Did she say anything to you?" Jenny and I had been nervous about bringing up this issue with Mom's minister because we weren't sure what his religious stance would be on this issue.

"Yes, she has also told me she doesn't want the stomach tube again."

Relief flooded through me. If it came down to it, the word of a minister would surely count for more than my own in case Dr. Adams wanted to insert a stomach tube again. "Don't worry," I said as I shook his hand goodbye. "We won't let them put in another feeding tube."

Then Rick arrived with his crew cut and boyish grin. My mother adored him. He was the person who found her in the hospital emergency room on Labor Day after her stroke, when the hospital wouldn't tell us anything on the phone. When Mom looked at him, her eyes shone, and a smile spread across her whole face. She reached out for his hands, held one, and stroked the other. She drank him in with her eyes. But even with Rick, she was unable to speak. She did try several times, but after sputtering a few words and finding it too hard, she contented herself with touching his shirt and stroking his hand.

Rick chatted animatedly with my mom, sharing news about his two daughters and the overtime he had worked that week at the utility company. She appeared fascinated by every word. She was enthralled, this woman who had shown no interest in my degrees, careers, international travel, or charity work! This woman who was supposed to be *my* mother! I was sick with jealousy. I could not bear to watch anymore. My heart was breaking.

"We're gonna go grab a coffee," I murmured to Rick. Luke and I slipped out the door as Rick nodded his head and kept on chatting with my mom.

On one level, I loved her enough to be happy she had friends in her life who cared about her and were able to make her happy. But on another level, a level so deep and primal it sometimes drowned out my rational mind, I wanted my mother to pay attention to *me*!

JOURNAL ENTRY 10-3

The nursing home called Jenny and told her that Mom was being released from the hospital today and returning to the nursing home. Transport was originally set for 2 p.m., but it was a little after six o'clock when she finally arrived at the nursing home. Mom had refused lunch in the hospital again, but I was optimistic that she would be much better when she returned to her familiar nursing-home room. I, myself, felt a surge of relief the minute I walked into the familiar carpeted lobby with the aviary in the corner.

As soon as Mom got into her bed, the staff brought in a tray of food. Her roommate, Sophie, was already asleep. Mom ate with gusto for several bites. She was so excited, she didn't wait for me to spoon-feed her but dug into the food with her hand. Of course, she began to cough because the muscles in her throat still didn't allow for proper swallowing. As soon as that happened, she pushed away her tray and wouldn't take another bite. I was sure she would feel better in the morning, though, waking up and having her own clothes to wear, her hearing aids in her ears, her own pictures on the walls, and her collection of lighthouses on the shelf. I certainly felt better just being in a room with cheerful yellow walls instead of that horribly bare, drab hospital room.

I had never thought the nursing home would feel so good to me, but I felt relief as I walked down the hall, greeting some of the staff by name. I popped into the dining room and joked with the residents. Several people asked about my mother. The nursing home was less than ideal, yes, but it was infinitely preferable to the sterile, hostile institution the hospital had been. I was glad Mom would be here instead of at the hospital when I would leave the next day.

This experience made it feel critical to Jenny and me that our mother never endure another hospital stay. The DNH was imperative to ensure she never would go through another hospitalization.

JOURNAL ENTRY 10-4

Pat, the daughter of another patient, mentioned that as a result of finding out that Jenny and I had gotten DNH paperwork for our mom, she had requested it for her mom too. Her mother had lived with Alzheimer's for years and was totally noncommunicative. The social worker at the nursing home gave Pat the form, which she filled out and handed in. Knowing you had to follow up on everything at the nursing home, a few weeks later,

Pat went to the shift nurse and asked if the DNH was in her mom's file.

The shift nurse said, "Yes, but it is completed incorrectly. The way this form is filled out means *you* will not be sent to a hospital!" Naturally, Pat got a different form and started the process again.

This worried me because the last time Jenny or I had seen our mom's DNH was in May, when Jenny had signed it. I asked at the last family meeting if the DNH was in Mom's file. The floor nurse and social worker made notes about this, then promised to check and get back to me. It had been over two weeks and no one had followed up, so I asked the social worker on my way past her office today. She said she would check and get back to me.

JOURNAL ENTRY 10-5

I arrived at the nursing home at about eleven thirty, and as usual, Mom was already in the dining room. *No* glasses, *no* hearing aids, hair unbrushed. We had switched her hospice aide to a morning time slot in the hopes that the hospice aide would pay more attention to getting her ready for the day. Obviously, this had been a misplaced hope.

Mom had only taken her first few bites of lunch when her floor nurse came in to say Mom's doctor, Dr. Adams, had arrived and wanted to look at her. She wheeled

Mom out of the dining room and into her room. I decided to tag along and have some contact with her doctor. The first thing I told him about was her hand. I pointed out that when I had visited her in May, she could still use most of it, but on this visit, it was curled up and useless. I said I wasn't sure whether it had been caused by arthritis or a stroke. I told him I had massaged it every day since then. I asked if he thought it was a good idea to continue the massage.

He acted as if he were seeing Mom's hand for the first time. As I talked to him about it, he tried to uncurl the fingers himself, then asked her to squeeze his hand. I was surprised that hospice hadn't communicated to him the state of Mom's hand. I had pointed it out to the hospice nurse shortly after I arrived in June, and I assumed she would tell the doctor about it.

He said the curling of the hand was the result of another stroke. He didn't think it would hurt for me to continue massaging her hand, but it wouldn't be helpful either. He listened to her lungs and heart. He moved her arms around. He looked at her skin. He made no comments during the exam but asked me if I had any specific questions for him.

I found it odd that he never ventured any big picture of Mom's condition. He never hazarded a forecast of her future. I, myself, had worked as an economist and as an attorney. It was my job in those professional roles to not only magnanimously offer to answer my clients' specific questions, but also to give them my general evaluation of the loan, contract, economy of Bulgaria, future price of petroleum, and so on. It was part of my job to give an overall impression, something like, "This contract looks good, but I'm concerned about your potential vulnerability if there should be a labor strike. We should add a clause about that." I would do this even if the client had not specifically raised the question of a labor strike himself!

My mother's doctor had not been forthcoming with us the entire time we dealt with him. I didn't know what questions to ask when we were living through my mother's time in the nursing home. But now, I asked the only question that really mattered to me, "Can you tell me what you see as her future?" I knew there were no guarantees. But in general, I hoped he could tell me if she would go along like this until she had a big stroke and died or if would there be constant deterioration.

He only shrugged his shoulders.

Later, Jenny, who handled the bills, told me he billed $100 for each of these visits to the nursing home. His office building was directly across the street from the nursing home, so there was no travel time involved. As my dad used to say, "Nice work if you can get it."

Jenny could legally handle Mom's bills because she and Mom had completed the form for a financial POA when Mom had her first TIA back in April.

Previous to her TIA, Mom had never told Jenny or me anything about her finances. Jenny knew Mom had an account at Bank of America because she had driven Mom there once. She didn't know if Mom had accounts at any other banks. We didn't know if she had any income or assets other than her pension and monthly social security checks. Even though Mom was eighty-eight when she had her first TIA, she had never made either of us POA, put us as signatories on her bank account, or told us if she had a will. In addition to these financial matters, we also didn't know if she had regularly visited any doctors other than Dr. Adams.

Mom had most certainly never discussed with us her wishes for end-of-life measures or funeral arrangements. Jenny and I were both painfully aware that our mother had relationships with people we didn't know, people who had sent her cards saying how much they loved her and what a great person she was. We had seen these cards in her apartment. It was possible that Mom had asked someone else to be her POA, and that would have been fine with us, but we wished we knew. While she was in the hospital in April, her mental condition was too disordered for her to answer such questions.

Immediately after her TIA, we had gone through her purse and the paperwork in her bureau drawers. Pineville needed to know if Mom had any supplemental insurance in addition to her Medicare. We found an envelope with this information on her dining room table. We were relieved to be able to tell them she had supplemental insurance.

But there were other issues. Rent needed to be paid on her apartment, and a utility bill had come in. We hated to bring up a subject she had avoided discussing our whole life—her finances—but it couldn't wait anymore. I broached the topic with her. "Mom, you have some bills that are due, like the rent on your apartment. Is there someone who can write checks and do your banking for you?"

"No," she replied.

"Mom, it would be really good if you would give permission for someone else to write checks or sign papers for you if you would get sick again and couldn't do it for yourself. Right now, it looks like you are going to get better again and go home, but just in case, Mom, *just in case* something else happened to you, and you went to the hospital again, it would be a good thing. Someone could do some of your business for you."

I had the financial POA paperwork in front of me. "Mom, here is a form that will let you give someone permission to do your banking and write checks for you. You can also revoke this paperwork if you want to later. I think it would be a really good idea to have this piece of paper signed. *Just in case.*"

Mom didn't say anything, so I pressed on. "Mom, I have a pen right here. I can write in someone's name. Would you like me to write in Jenny's name or someone else's?"

"Jenny," she whispered.

"Okay, Mom, that's great." I wrote in my sister's name, checked the applicable boxes, got two aides to be witnesses, and had my mom sign it before she could change her mind. I had her sign two copies so my sister would have an easier time of it. Mom's signature was shaky, but she was still able to sign. I heaved a big sigh of relief.

And that was how it came about that we had a financial POA.

JOURNAL ENTRY 10-6

I decided I'd better check to see if they had the DNH for Mom in her official nursing-home file.

I noticed Mom's floor nurse today was the same one who was at the last family meeting at the nursing home. "Diana," I said brightly. "Do you remember, at my mom's last family meeting, I asked if her DNH was in order? I was wondering if you had a chance to check on that yet?"

Diana said, "I'll check right now." She leafed through a thick, three-ring binder about my mom and said, "Here it is, right here in her chart!"

I was close enough to read it. "Diana, it isn't signed by the director of nursing. Is that okay?"

"Oh darn," she said. "I have a minute. I'll go check on that right now."

This annoyed me because it only needed three signatures: Jenny's (as health care POA for my mom), Mom's doctor, and the director of nursing. Jenny and the doctor had signed it on June 5. It was now July 11.

Diana toddled back, all bright-eyed and bushy-tailed. "I have it all signed now."

"Can I take it and make a copy?" I asked deferentially.

Diana ripped the carbon copy off the original and handed it to me with a flourish. I was very happy to have that DNH signed, sealed, and filed. I left with a copy in my purse!

JOURNAL ENTRY 10-7

Jenny called me on the phone. "The social worker came up to me while I had Mom in the lobby, there in front of that window in the front she likes best. The social worker said, 'I was looking at your mom's DNH, and I don't know if it is really the right one. You got that form from the hospice nurse, and it is different from the one we use here at the nursing home. I'll print off another DNH form for you to sign.'"

Jenny and I were old veterans of this kind of aggravation. We *liked* to think we just rolled with the punches and let this bureaucratic incompetence roll off our backs. But still, this really annoyed us.

First of all, the hospice we were using was one of the three hospices *recommended* by this nursing home. It wasn't like we were using fly-by-night hospice.

Second, this form was initially handed to the nursing home on May 5, and no one bothered to scrutinize it until July 11 or 12—and only then because I had pursued it. Would they really make my poor, little mother go back to the hospital, even though her daughter, doctor, and the nursing home's *own* director of nursing had signed the form? We were incredulous.

Jenny, of course, signed the new form. But we wondered who would bother to get it to Mom's doctor for his signature. He wouldn't be back to the nursing home for at least a month or so since he had just been there last week, and there was no telling if either of us would be there when he did.

In the meantime, would they actually drag Mom back to the hospital if she were to develop pneumonia?

JOURNAL ENTRY 10-8

I noticed that Mom looked skinny. She used to look fat in the middle because of her diaper. But recently, she looked so skinny around the waist that I pulled down her slacks to make sure she had a diaper on. I wondered how much she weighed now. I'd asked the floor nurse a few days ago, but she had been too busy, and I told her there was no rush. Residents were supposed to be weighed on the first of the month. So today, I asked again about Mom's weight, and the nurse said she would get back to me.

JOURNAL ENTRY 10-9

Jenny had a friendly chat with Mom's floor nurse and mentioned we were wondering about Mom's weight. The floor nurse opened Mom's chart and said, "Hmmm, they didn't weigh your mom in July." She did give Jenny the weights for May and June. Mom had weighed 112 pounds on June 1.

JOURNAL ENTRY 10-10

Jenny and I had taken the day off to visit Longwood Gardens. I didn't get to the nursing home until nearly five o'clock. The first thing I did was to seek out the 3 p.m. to 11 p.m. floor nurse. I asked her if Mom had been weighed. She checked her notes and told me my mom weighed ninety-six pounds.

"That's impossible, Phyllis!" I sputtered. "That just can't be. That would mean she lost sixteen pounds in a little over two months. With me and Jenny feeding her twice a day, every day! This couldn't be possible! Do you think someone could have made a mistake when they weighed her?"

Strategic error on my part! Never question the competence of the staff!

Phyllis puffed herself up and replied, "I weighed her myself. She definitely weighed ninety-six pounds. And there is no record of her weight since June 1."

How could this be so difficult? It wasn't as though my mother had a rare disease, and I was begging for them to create a cure. This was just about weighing a person, for crying out loud! This wasn't rocket science! How could this be *too much* to ask? And given that all the staff knew, or should have known, about Mom's ongoing swallowing difficulties, her weight was critical data to prove whether she was taking in enough nutrition by mouth.

After I had calmed down, I went and found Mom. She had already eaten her mashed potatoes. I gave her a cup of pudding and showed her the present I brought her from Longwood Gardens. Then I washed her face, grabbed her afghan from the closet, and wheeled her outside.

"Mom, did your friend Charles come to visit you today?" Charles was her friend from church who normally visited her on Monday, Wednesday, and Friday mornings. But he had been on vacation all summer. This was the first day he was scheduled to be back. Jenny and I had banked on his return when we planned our outing.

I was stunned by her response. She spoke in complete sentences! Her story went something like this: "Charles and his son went on a hike in the mountains. It was very hard. Going down was really hard. They fell. They had to hold on to rocks."

Her narration was slow and painstaking. But I hadn't had to prompt her with more questions, and I could understand every word. I was nearly in tears because I was so happy. How had this miracle occurred? I had done some research on stroke recovery and aphasia after it became obvious that her doctors were not going to tell us anything about her condition. What I had read was that patients make the most significant recovery during the first six months after a stroke. It seemed to me that therapists adjusted their expectations of recovery accordingly. But here, it was nearly a year to the day since her big stroke, and she was just now uttering her first complete sentences. I say to others, "Don't let that six-month guideline limit your efforts for rehabilitation!"

JOURNAL ENTRY 10-11

I was still worried about finding out Mom's actual weight. If she had really lost sixteen pounds, then something profoundly wrong was going on. I resolved to stick at this until I got her weighed again.

Oh God, I love her so much. How will I ever drive away on Saturday?

FOR THE RECORD

A New York study of forty-three thousand nursing-home residents found that 61 percent had do-not-resuscitate (DNR) orders, but only 6 percent had DNH orders.[43]

The following information on paperwork is general information only and is not intended to serve as legal advice. Paperwork varies by state, so you need to find out which forms are legal in your state as well as what is required for witnesses or notarization. Some states may require both. Consult a licensed attorney for any questions you have!

Do Not Resuscitate. A DNR is a legal order that indicates the person does not want to undergo CPR or advanced cardiac life support if they were to stop breathing. Even with a DNR, a patient can still receive chemotherapy, antibiotics, dialysis, and other treatments.[44]

Do Not Hospitalize. A DNH order can take two forms, and it is up to the patient to decide which she would prefer. One is an absolute ban on being sent to a hospital for any reason whatsoever. The other form can spell out specific reasons they would consent to being hospitalized—e.g., in case of profuse bleeding or severe pain—and in the absence of those specific reasons, they will not be hospitalized. It is important to remember that if the language for exceptions to the DNH order is vague, then medical professionals will fall back on their default choice of always hospitalizing a patient if there is any doubt.[45]

Patient Charts. What I didn't know at the time of my mother's illness is that my sister, because she held Mom's health care POA, had a legal right to see our mother's charts in the nursing home. This right is codified in the federal regulations. This regulation states that a resident or her legal representative "has the right of access to all records, including current clinical records within twenty-four hours (excluding weekends and holidays) of an oral or written request." Further, photocopies of those records may be purchased upon request with two days of notice.[46]

Power of Attorney. It is important to follow up and make sure the health care POA is in the nursing home's files and that you keep at least one additional copy of this form in a safe place. Please be aware that a financial POA is different from a health care POA; a POA designated as financial does not have the right to see medical records unless the financial POA specifically conveys a health care POA.

Weight. Nursing homes are required to weigh residents every month. It is one way to determine if a patient, especially one on a feeding tube, is getting sufficient nutrition.[47]

TIPS

- Choose a health care POA now if you haven't already. Make sure the form is signed and your health care POA is willing to take on this responsibility. Have the form witnessed and notarized if required by your state. Keep one copy yourself and give copies to your health care POA, doctor, and hospital.
- Execute an advance medical directive as a favor to yourself and your family. Directives are well known, yet only 38 percent of all Americans have one.[48]
- Review your paperwork once each year.
- Be aware that if someone dials 911 for help, advance medical directives might be ignored. This is because the duty of a first responder is to attempt to resuscitate the patient and transport them to the hospital.[49]
- Follow-up with nursing-home staff regarding weight checks. Nursing homes certified by the Centers for Medicare & Medicaid Services (CMS) must regularly report information about each patient, including the percentage of long-term residents who have lost 5 percent (or more) of their weight in the past month or 10 percent over the past six months. Weight loss can indicate that the resident is sick, depressed, has a situation that makes it difficult to eat, isn't being fed properly, or lives in a nursing home that offers poor nutrition. Weight loss can affect the dosage of prescription medication and/or put a resident at risk for pressure ulcers.[50]

CHAPTER 11
More Frustrations

JOURNAL ENTRY 11-1

Last night, I laid out Mom's pink pedal pushers and a pink top for her to wear today. Whoever dressed Mom this morning used the pink clothes but chose red socks even though she had pink ones in the drawer. A year ago, Mom would have caused a fuss about the choice of socks, would even have demanded a different color. Now, she seemed oblivious to this fashion faux pas.

Jenny and I got to the nursing home together a little after noon, and Mom was already in the dining room. Even though there were two aides at a table of five patients, a good ratio, Mom had big globs of mashed potatoes on her face. She was feeding herself. I didn't expect the aides to do anything anymore, so I wasn't surprised they hadn't wiped her face. It probably wasn't in their job description to do it.

After lunch, we took her out in the courtyard for a little variation. I stuck my bare foot in her lap, and she pretended to tickle the bottom of my foot as I pretended to laugh. This made her laugh for real, which made me happy for real.

We brought her into her room a little before two o'clock, and her hospice nurse, Laura, was there talking to Mom's roommate. Laura told us Mom's cough must be better because "no one had noted her cough on the chart."

I was dumbfounded. Not because no one had noted she was coughing, but because Laura would conclude that the absence of information on the chart meant the condition didn't exist. Didn't she know better? I assured her that Mom had been coughing every day.

When I got back at five o'clock, Mom was in bed and her supper tray was on the rolling bedside table. She had an oxygen cannula in her nose. I fed her the small container of cottage cheese I had brought with me and about half the mashed potatoes and gravy on her plate. She asked for pudding and ate most of that. I noticed she had only one hearing aid in her ear, so I searched around her clothes and blankets, but I couldn't find the other one. We had gone to such great lengths to get the hearing aids replaced and had them add strings with alligator clips to clip onto her clothes. How could *one* hearing aid be missing?

I went down to the nurses' station where a different floor nurse was on duty. I was positively weary of the frequent staff changes at this place. If I couldn't keep track of them, then what chance did my mom, or any of the other patients, have of keeping track of staff names and roles?

I introduced myself as Hazel's daughter and asked what Mom's pulse ox—heart rate and oxygen saturation—had been earlier in the day to prompt the oxygen use. She ignored my question but went down to Mom's room and took a reading right then. It was ninety-four. That was a decent reading when you'd been breathing in the air from the room, but from the machine? I really didn't know. The good news was that the floor nurse had found Mom's one hearing aid in a box on the med cart. *Why* one hearing aid and not the other one? How would that happen? The strings on her hearing aids are quite visible as they are pink! Just a mystery.

The floor nurse also told me that the hospice nurse had left a note saying Mom was to be given cough medicine each evening between 8 p.m. and 9 p.m.

I said, "That's good because my mom has been coughing in the evenings."

"I know," she replied. "I have requested a chest X-ray be done for her."

How did we get from two o'clock, when the hospice nurse assumed Mom didn't have a cough because it wasn't noted, to six o'clock the same day, when the floor nurse said she had requested a chest X-ray? If I hadn't been there to witness this myself, I would not have believed it.

JOURNAL ENTRY 11-2

Wow! I was so thrilled today when I walked into Mom's room and saw a child's sippy cup on her tray table. Oh, how grand! Now she could take a drink of her thickened juice without spilling it all down the front of her shirt. I took the sippy cup in my hands and mimed using it. Mom watched me, her eyes big without her glasses. Even a plastic sippy cup was a little heavy for her to handle, but we were both determined she would master it. It would still be difficult to find someone to open the foil on the top of the nectar cup and pour it into her sippy cup, but this was progress. More importantly, the sippy cup showed that someone cared.

I didn't know who to thank for this blessed innovation. I went to the kitchen and asked, but no one seemed to know anything about it. I called Charles and asked him, but he hadn't provided it either. It was another mystery, but one I was very grateful for.

JOURNAL ENTRY 11-3

Mom's sippy cup honeymoon came to an abrupt end today. Each day for the past three days, a clean sippy cup had miraculously appeared on Mom's tray table before I arrived there in the morning. But this afternoon, the floor nurse happened to enter Mom's room, a rare occurrence. She spied that sippy cup and blew a gasket.

"How dare you bring a sippy cup for your mom?" she demanded in a loud voice.

I tried to explain. "I didn't bring it! It just appeared here. I don't know how it got here."

"Oh no, no, *no*! You or your sister *must* have brought that sippy cup in. There is no other way it could have gotten here. Your mother still has swallowing issues. A sippy cup is *not* permitted for your mother. I can't believe you just went and did this without even asking."

"I. Did. Not. *Do*. This!" Oh my God, how could this woman be so angry with me for something I did not do? I didn't ask for this. I never even thought of it. But why wouldn't she believe me when I said I didn't bring the sippy cup?

The floor nurse continued to excoriate me for several more minutes until I finally burst into tears and dashed to my car. I called Jenny and told her what happened.

After that, I didn't want to be in the nursing home at the same time as that floor nurse, but I had to go back. My poor, little mother hadn't been entirely tracking our conversation, but she could tell from the tone and volume of the shouting that I had done something to make the nurse very angry. And Mom would be worried.

JOURNAL ENTRY 11-4

Today, I saw Mom's floor nurse coming toward me in the dining room. It was like watching a tornado beeline toward me—and I had no basement to run to for shelter. For a fleeting moment, I thought about hiding under the table. She asked me to come out into the hall with her.

Oh Lord, I wondered, *am I going to be banished from the nursing home for the crime of bringing a sippy cup to my mother when I didn't even do it? Don't I have a right to an attorney? Heck, I* am *an attorney! If the nursing home has managed to cow me to this extent, how must the helpless residents feel?*

The floor nurse then proceeded to explain that one of the CNAs had admitted to bringing my mother a sippy cup. She had seen how much my mother struggled to use a spoon or do anything with her hands. She thought the sippy cup would be helpful.

Mystery solved. I was off the hook, but that nurse did not have the decency to apologize for accusing me of something I hadn't done.

Jenny and I both had been worn down to less than nubs from the ongoing stress of trying to get the nursing home to perform routine tasks—brush Mom's hair, clean her teeth, put her glasses on, turn her hearing aids on (and not lose them), and wash her hands more often than once a week. Yet, we still struggled with all our might to be courteous and treat the staff decently. But this was the last straw for me. I didn't know how much more of this I could take.

By and large, we didn't think the staff was evil. We knew they were overworked and underpaid. But they were all we had to depend upon. I didn't know who to contact, how to frame my requests, or what could be done to improve the quality of my mother's life within the very narrow confines of her physical limitations. She couldn't walk, turn over, move from her bed to her wheelchair, or propel her wheelchair once she was in it. She was utterly dependent on others.

It was obvious to me and Jenny that, without us to advocate for her, she wouldn't get the tiny assistances that *would* help her, such as opening nectar or yogurt cups, or even the larger, legally mandated actions, such as a monthly weigh-in. These were acts of care we felt we shouldn't have had to manipulate the staff to provide for Mom. We were fresh out of strategies to cope with this mountain of thoughtlessness.

JOURNAL ENTRY 11-5

Mom was agitated when I walked in this morning. She kept saying, "In my room, in my room." I set about guessing her problem by pointing to items in her room. "Do you want to look at your cards? Do you want this afghan?"

"No, no, no!" she wailed.

She was as defenseless as a kitten and, in my eyes, just as adorable. "Is it something already in your room?"

"No."

"Is it something that *was* in your room but isn't now?"

"Yeth. At night."

"*What?* Something comes into your room at night?" I couldn't believe it.

"He sits there."

I won't bore you with how long it took to guess and piece together her little story. But apparently, she thought someone was coming into her room at night, sitting in her visitor chair next to the bed, and staring at her. Jenny and I conferred and quickly agreed that Mom must have been dreaming this because who on earth would come into her room after lights out, sit in the chair, and stare at her?

We sought to assure her that no one was coming into her room. We told her she was safe where she was, but she wasn't buying it.

In the morning, I went to watch the group exercise class Mom participated in a few mornings each week. Her days of full-on physical therapy in hopes of walking again were over after a few heady weeks of hope. The wheelchair-confined residents were urged to reach their arms up as though they were hanging up clothes or picking apples. My mom tried, but she couldn't even get her arms up to shoulder height. Mom didn't even try to pretend she was kicking a soccer ball. I didn't blame her.

This afternoon, I rolled her outside so we could talk and sing. Even though the occupational therapy and physical therapy had fizzled out, I remembered the speech therapist had always wanted her to practice saying k sounds and was determined to work with her on this. I don't think the speech therapist ever told me why the k sound was important, but I figured it couldn't hurt to work on it. My husband had taken a job in Copenhagen, Denmark, and when I went there to visit him, I took several pictures and organized them into a book to show them to Mom. I could tell she really wasn't tracking where Denmark was, but she obediently looked at the pictures. And when I urged her to repeat "Copenhagen" and "Denmark" while looking at the pictures, she had lots of experience making the k sound.

JOURNAL ENTRY 11-6

I brought Mom a small bouquet of flowers when I went to the nursing home this morning. Spring was definitely in the air, and I looked forward to wheeling Mom outside to look at the daffodils in the yard.

At her doorway, I stopped in shock. Her hair was hacked off on one side of her head! She had only about two inches of hair on that one side. I stepped closer and saw the eyebrow on that same side of her face had also been cut off. The other eyebrow was intact.

This completely blew my mind. Someone must have come into her room in the middle of the night. There were only three possibilities as to the visitor's identity: another patient, a staff member, or an outside person. The idea that another patient could possibly have had access to scissors really frightened me.

I reported this to the nurses' station. "Debbie, you know how my mom said that someone was coming into her room at night, but we just couldn't believe her? Well, last night, someone came into her room and *cut her hair!*"

Debbie scoffed and said this wasn't possible.

"Come with me!" I commanded and hustled back to my mom's room. For once, a staff person responded immediately!

Debbie and I stood by my mother's bed and surveyed her hair. Debbie shook her head slowly and said, "I know who did this. Don't worry, it won't happen again."

Even though I later asked her a few more times whom she believed the culprit to be, Debbie would never tell me. I asked primarily because my mother continued to fret about it, and I didn't blame her one bit. She was completely defenseless there in her bed; she couldn't even yell or roll onto her side to evade the scissors.

As far as we knew, no one came in and cut my mom's hair again. Whether or not that person ever came in and stared at her while she was sleeping, we have no way of knowing.

REPORTS FROM OTHERS

You could hear the anger in Betty's voice when she recounted her story. "They never came on time to give my mother-in-law her albuterol treatments. She went for five days without getting her prescribed albuterol treatments before she told me about it. When the staff was told about this, they didn't say they were sorry or give a reason, just tried to pass the buck. They asked her, 'Are you *sure* you didn't have it last night?'" When Betty asked to check the chart to see if the albuterol had been logged, they made her sign releases. Then they told her it would take a week to get the chart. That was over a year ago, and to this day, they have never been able to see those, or any, of her mother-in-law's charts. Because she hadn't gotten her albuterol breathing treatments, she wound up being sent to the hospital. At the hospital, they said she had pneumonia in both lungs.

Betty's mother-in-law also had MRSA. The facility told Betty and her husband that MRSA was not a big deal because "everybody" tests positive for MRSA.

Nancy was a professional occupational therapist for decades. She had a dear friend with no family who went into a nursing home. Nancy visited her several times a week on a regular basis. What she saw there appalled her. "My friend had heart problems and was supposed to have her legs elevated. There is an attachment for leg rests for the wheelchair, and they rarely would put those leg rests on her wheelchair. As a result, her feet were down to the floor and would drag a little on the floor as the wheelchair went forward. They would not let her walk to the dining room even though, at first, she *could* have. The reason they wouldn't let her walk was because it took more time than putting her in a wheelchair and wheeling her there. It just annoyed me so much because she needed to be encouraged to keep walking for as long as she could!"

She saw a whole array of problems. It annoyed Nancy to see the aides doing things for patients that the patients could have done for themselves, leading to an atrophy of skills and muscles. An example of this was a patient who'd had a stroke. "The stroke patient received [occupational therapy] to learn to dress herself with one hand. But the aides thought it took her too long, so the CNA would just dress her each day. And, of course, she eventually lost the ability to do this herself."

Even though Samantha's husband had passed away two years ago, she still sounded extremely frustrated when she recounted, "They put diapers on him immediately when he entered the nursing home. But he didn't need diapers; he was still continent. He felt very humiliated by wearing diapers and kept asking why he had to wear them when he could still get to the bathroom." Staff had diapered him so they were covered, in case they didn't answer his call button in a timely fashion.

Claire Johnson fumed when she remembered, "Mom didn't want to hurt anybody's feelings. She didn't want to get anybody in trouble. She didn't want to make waves because she felt vulnerable and at their mercy. The key staff *knew* she didn't want to get anybody in trouble and took advantage of it. When my mom got a wound on her leg that wasn't healing [cellulitis], the nurse said, 'Yeah, your feet are swollen.' This was on a Friday, and they did nothing. I had to take her to the hospital the following week. I went on a rant with a nurse about the wound, and that nurse never went back to see if my mom was okay. This is just one example of us complaining and them not doing anything. They had certainly seen the wound when they were dressing her. The nurse lied directly to my face, telling me she had checked my mother's leg when she had not."

Claire Johnson continued, "A few months later, my mom fell and broke her knee. They did nothing. They visually looked at her knee and said, 'It is fine.' I went in two days later, and her knee was swollen up bigger than a grapefruit. When she had an X-ray, it showed she had two broken bones. Just getting the X-ray was an ordeal. Her facility was supposed to transport her to the clinic."

Claire went directly to the place where the X-ray was to happen to meet her mother there. The nursing home her mom was in had two vans, but as it turned out, both were broken, and they didn't have a driver anyway. A CNA going off duty put Claire's mom in her own compact car. This was agonizing for a woman with broken bones in her leg! Getting her out of the car to get the X-ray was even worse.

"It was at this time that I discovered that the nursing home had changed her medications arbitrarily," Claire explained. "A staff member had started giving my mom a high dose of aspirin for pain relief for her knee. This would have been okay except for the fact that my mom had been on blood thinners for years. The nursing home didn't catch this; it was the doctor at urgent care who figured it out."

FOR THE RECORD

I have lumped several stories together under the heading of "More Frustrations" for lack of a better unifying topic. I use the term "frustration" in this chapter to refer to any actions, or lack thereof, that just aren't right. Whether or not they rise to the legal definition of "negligence" is open for discussion.

"Negligence" is a legal term that means an entity, such as a nursing home, had a duty to someone, such as a resident, but they breached that duty and that breach caused harm to the person they had a duty to. The harms cited most frequently in lawsuits against nursing homes are death, bedsores, dehydration, weight loss, and emotional distress. A single instance of a mistake or oversight will not usually rise to the level of negligence; there must be a pattern of actions or omissions.

Neglect and abuse in nursing homes are more common than the general public would like to acknowledge, and they are getting worse. The US Government Accountability Office (GAO) reported to the US Senate Committee on Finance in 2019 that abuse in nursing homes had more than doubled between 2013 and 2017. The greatest increase was in actual harm and immediate jeopardy. This abuse is significantly underreported.[51]

According to a study by the National Research Council, only one in fourteen possible cases of abuse are reported; that is about six thousand cases not reported in 2016. Why are these abuse offenses underreported? First, many residents feel embarrassed to have had this happen to them and do not wish to go public with their shame. Second, there is often a fear that there will be reprisals from the nursing-home staff. I remember how my mother referred to the staff as her "guards" and never wanted to do anything to make them angry. Third, many residents have verbal or mental impairments that make communicating this information to an outside person difficult, if not impossible.[52]

If you have encountered activity (or lack thereof) that you believe falls under the legal definition of "negligence," you need to think about whether you have proof of the nursing home's negligence. It is possible that your loved one will encounter not just negligence but also abuse in a nursing home. The distinction between the two often comes down to the intention of the one causing the harm. A congressional study of nursing homes from January 1999 to January 2001 reported that 30 percent of nursing homes had been cited for almost nine thousand instances of abuse or neglect or both.[53]

Should you seek legal advice, an attorney who decides to take your case is likely to do so on a contingency basis, meaning they take a percentage of the amount you are awarded.

It is estimated that about 90 percent of nursing-home lawsuits are settled out of court. A few examples of out-of-court settlements are $65,000 in Pennsylvania for a fall that resulted in amputation of a leg; $4.5 million in Oklahoma for a woman trapped in a walk-in freezer; and $5.2 million in Arkansas for a death due to sepsis. You should be aware that there is a time limit between when an action (or lack of action) occurred and when you can file a lawsuit. This is referred to as the "statute of limitations." This varies by state and can be as brief as one year—Kentucky, Louisiana, and Tennessee—or as long as six years—Maine, North Dakota.[54]

There was an effort by the Trump administration to make it impossible for nursing-home residents or their representatives to sue a nursing home for negligence. This would have allowed nursing homes to require a signed form agreeing to arbitration rather than a court case as a condition before admission.[55]

In July, 2019, this regulation—requiring a signature waiving the right to bring a lawsuit but instead agreeing to submit grievances to arbitration—was rolled back by CMS. The new rule, CMS-3342-F, prohibits any long-term care facility from *requiring* such an arbitration agreement, but they still are permitted.[56]

It had not occurred to me that there was a term for the other person who had stared at my mother while she slept, and who ultimately cut her hair and eyebrow. It was only while researching for this book that I encountered the term "resident-to-resident elder mistreatment." In an analysis of the rights of nursing-home residents under the Nursing Home Reform Act of 1987 and the subsequent 2016 revisions published in *National Academy of Elder Law Attorneys*, I learned that "resident-to-resident elder mistreatment (RREM) is 'negative physical, sexual, or verbal interactions between long-term care residents that, in a community setting, would likely be construed as unwelcome and have high potential to cause physical or psychological distress in the recipient.'" Further, this behavior is "common" based on reports from nursing-home staff. The majority of the RREM is verbal, but there also have been reports of physical and sexual RREM.[57]

The article also explains, "Although seemingly harmless in some cases, [RREM] can have devastating consequences. The frailty of many nursing home residents makes minor incidents potentially catastrophic. Residents who suffer from dementia may act out violently. Sadly, there are multiple examples of residents being injured or killed by another resident. A resident who is violent must be safely supervised to ensure that he or she does not harm himself or herself or others. Failure to provide necessary supervision for a violent resident can lead to injury and even death of the resident, other residents, staff members, or visitors." In retrospect, I do not think the nursing-home staff took my mother's report of this behavior seriously enough.[58]

TIPS

- Always double-check the medications even though it is the staff's job, and they are theoretically checking charts and medications daily. As Betty reminds, "Every time my mom had a decline, we were able to track it back and find there were errors in the medication being given to her."
- Keep your options open. Do not, at the time of admission, sign an agreement not to bring a lawsuit against a nursing home.
- Be aware of signs of possible nursing-home abuse: bleeding, bruising negative changes in behavior, unexplained sickness, and infection.[59]
- Err on the side of believing a report of negligence or abuse coming from your loved one who lives in a nursing home. Do a little detective work, if you can, to figure out what is actually occurring. If the complaint turns out to be unfounded, you can simply reassure the person that the problem is not really as bad as they think. If the complaint is, indeed, a reality, then you can take steps to advocate on their behalf.
- Reach out to your local ombudsman if you have a problem concerning the care, or lack thereof, in a nursing home. The Long-Term Care Ombudsman Program was created in 1972 by the Older Americans Act. Nationally, the program has 8,700 volunteers and more than 1,300 paid

staff. They regularly visit and investigate resident welfare in nursing homes, board-and-care facilities, and assisted-living communities. There should be contact information for your local ombudsman posted on the wall of the nursing home. If you don't see it there, you can go to their website, https://ltcombudsman.org/, to learn more about the services provided and locate an ombudsman near you.

CHAPTER 12
Staff

I left Pineville a little before four o'clock and came back at 5:30 p.m. When I arrived, the floor nurse was trying to put the oxygen cannula into my mom's nose. Mom was flailing weakly around in bed, saying, "No, no, no."

"Hi, Debbie," I said while reaching out to calm my mother. "Is her pulse ox low?"

"Your mother just needs some oxygen to be more comfortable. But she doesn't seem to want it."

"Well, what was the reading on her pulse ox?" I asked.

"I didn't take it," she admitted.

Staff are expected to check her pulse ox once each shift, but I suspected this rule was not followed routinely.

Debbie added, "She told the aide she was having trouble breathing."

Just then, the aide walked in. She was one I had seen occasionally but not often enough to memorize her name. Debbie asked the aide what Mom had said. The aide, whose English was not very good, was struggling to recall what Mom had said when Mom burst out, "Compacted! I told her I'm compacted."

I looked down at her. The head of her bed was elevated as always, but she had slid down the slope of the mattress. There, her torso crumpled up in the valley where the top half of the mattress intersected with the flat, bottom half.

I understood and asked. "Mom, do you want to be pulled up?"

"Yeth," she murmured with relief.

Debbie and I pulled Mom up on the mattress, stretching out her torso in the process. "Do you feel better now?" I asked.

"Yeth," she said. The nurse and I smiled at each other as the nurse and aide left.

JOURNAL ENTRY 12-2

I didn't know whether to scream or cry. I knew by now that either response would be ineffective. But honestly, how many times had I walked into Mom's room in the last year to find a cup of nectar or yogurt sitting on her tray table with a plastic spoon sitting beside it and the lid still on top of the container? Anyone could see that my mother's hands were incapable of removing a *lid* from the top of a yogurt cup. If you put a plastic spoon in her hand and opened the container for her, she had a good chance of getting some yogurt into her mouth. But if the lid had not been removed, the container may as well have been on Mars for all the good it would do my mom.

I had pointed this out to every aide I could identify who did this. But the stream of replacement aides presented me with an ongoing river of new names, faces, and native languages.

When I tell people outside the nursing home about this particular frustration, they always tell me, "Oh, those aides are so pressed for time. They have so much work to do. You can't expect them to open a yogurt cup." I am here to tell you I have timed myself to see how long it actually takes. It takes *six seconds* to open a yogurt or nectar cup!

The first eleven chapters of this book provide numerous instances where our problems in the nursing home could have been prevented, or solved, if there had been sufficient staff. I won't repeat those stories in this chapter. It is obvious that staff, and the lack thereof, impacts all aspects of life in a nursing home.

REPORTS FROM OTHERS

Patricia, who was a CNA, offered her perspective on CNAs working in nursing homes. "Here in North Carolina, I would say the CNAs in this community are those who are coming from a lower income level. That's valuable to know because a lot of CNAs are not caring for themselves, so how can they care for others? As for most of the CNAs I worked with, caring for others was not their passion. They didn't enjoy doing it. It was just a job. There's no self-care—you can see it in their bodies and in the way they talk to people. I believe if they can't help themselves, they really can't help others."

Patricia shared with me about her CNA training and its limitations. "No one taught me to prepare a body for burial or how to put a hearing aid in someone's ear. Most of my training was about the things we had to do, and not do, to avoid being sued. Changing a urinary bag was not taught. Lifting someone out of a wheelchair *was* taught." No one taught her about swallowing issues that require food and liquids to be thickened before giving them to patients. There is such a scarcity of CNAs that the only reason a CNA ever got fired, that she knew of, was for letting a patient fall.

Patricia recommended there be staff reviews and feedback given to CNAs. She was never given either. She never had any in-service training during her five years working as a CNA. Her caseload was typically twelve residents. She explained, "In that line of work, it is easy for someone to forget that their patient is a human being, and there is love and joy still left in that person. It is too easy to just get caught up in getting them dressed and fed. I wish someone had trained me a little better so I could have been more empathetic. It is so sad. The people I came in contact with, especially those without family, that was so sad to see. That was the hardest part for me."

Patricia concluded, "You have to *think* from someone else's perspective. I think this is something that CNAs should be trained for, to think from the perspective of the patient because it is not an assembly line. You need to get outside of yourself and think from the other person's perspective."

Andrea, who has worked as a CNA as well as in other capacities in long-term care facilities, told me, "I know what it is like when you are a CNA, and you are trying desperately to get everything done in a short amount of time. But I also sympathize with the patients who need these little things, like taking the foil off the nectar cup. It would only take a second or two to do that, but they are not thinking from the patient's perspective. They are just thinking, 'What do I have to get done?' A CNA would have to put herself into the framework of the person who can't move or communicate."

Betty remembered her CNA training. "We were familiarized with things such as equipment. We were never taught about people who had swallowing issues who needed thickener in their liquids. We were never taught to look for a sign or symbol in a patient's room that indicated 'nothing by mouth.'" She continued, "CNAs are really left to the wolves. They come in with good hearts. Once they are in a facility, they see what's wrong, and they are completely helpless to do anything about it. And if they report it, they lose their jobs."

THINGS TO KEEP IN MIND

Hierarchy. The hierarchy of nursing-home staff, based solely on my observation, is this: at the top is a director of nursing. This person is always an RN. Medicare mandates, due to the Nursing Home Reform Law of 1987, at least one RN be on the physical premises for eight hours per day, seven days per week.[60] The director of nursing at Pineville was a very nice and friendly person on the few occasions I saw her. She was almost always in her office, not on the floor with the patients.

In the middle of the hierarchy is the licensed practical nurse (LPN). This is the person I refer to most often as the "floor nurse." She was always my go-to person when I had a question about my mom's care or paperwork. Medicare mandates at least one LPN on duty 24/7.

Then there are the CNAs, whom I also refer to as "aides." The CNAs do the lion's share of all direct, hands-on patient care. The CNAs change diapers, turn patients who are bedridden, give baths, dress and undress patients, move patients out of (and into) bed, and help them eat. They are risking their backs every day on the job. For all this, the median annual CNA salary, according to the US Bureau of Labor Statistics in 2018, is around $26,500 but varies by geographic location. As a point of comparison, licensed practical nurses have an annual median salary of $44,090.[61]

The training of CNAs varies wildly and can range from four to twelve weeks. Prospective CNAs can take programs through community colleges, hospitals, the American Red Cross, vocational schools, and even in some high schools. It used to be common for nursing homes to offer their own CNA training programs, but fewer and fewer nursing homes offer this training each year. Each state sets its own rules for certification, and some states require periodic recertification.

Understaffing. Understaffing is a huge issue in nursing-home care. It is estimated that about 95 percent of long-term care facilities are understaffed.[62] Understaffing is not only a strain on the staff members, but it is also a major contributor to negligence of patients. Studies have shown that understaffing leads to a higher risk of malnutrition, weight loss, bedsores, falls, and infections among the residents.[63]

The Centers for Medicare & Medicaid Services do not mandate a specific caseload for CNAs or a minimum amount of time for each patient to receive direct care each day. They are only required to "provide sufficient staff and services." The centers have said, however, that the preferred minimum staffing level would give each nursing-home resident three hours of total staff time each day, broken down into two hours from a CNA and one hour from an LPN.[64]

An informal poll of thousands of nursing-home staff found that caseloads were unrealistic. In Ohio, it was reported that one nurse had thirty-two patients while each CNA had sixteen. In Illinois, those ratios were thirty-three per nurse and seventeen patients per CNA. In Nebraska, the caseload was even heavier—sixty patients per nurse and twenty per CNA.[65]

Patricia, a former CNA, thought lowering the CNA caseload is the only realistic way to solve the problem. "If you can keep the numbers down, then you get quality care." She estimated a reasonable caseload would be "six to eight residents if those residents are mobile. 'Mobile' meaning capable of getting up and walking on their own. For immobile patients, the maximum would be five. Six would be pushing it." She, herself, typically had twelve patients in her caseload.

If you want to do the math on patient caseloads for a CNA, begin with an eight-hour workday and subtract one hour—half-hour lunch and two fifteen-minute breaks. That leaves seven hours. Subtract another hour for 7 a.m. to 3 p.m. and 3 p.m. to 11 p.m. shifts for mealtime—delivering trays to those in bed, getting patients to the dining room and lined up with the right beverages and cutlery, and keeping a watchful eye that those with special health diets don't get the wrong food, and so on. This leaves six hours of time divided by twelve patients. That equals to an average of thirty minutes per day, per patient, for direct care—getting dressed, changing diapers, looking for eyeglasses, and more. You can see why the aides are rushed off their feet and don't have time to figure out what a patient is trying to say if she has speech difficulties!

State Mandates. According to a study by the CMS, "the key to improving nursing home staffing levels is increasing state standards. A study by Charlene Harrington, professor of Nursing and Sociology at the University of California, San Francisco, found that states with the highest standards for nursing staff levels are the only states where nursing homes have enough staff to prevent serious safety violations."[66] In the absence of a federal mandate for CNA caseloads, several states have enacted their own regulations.

Reporting Hours. Until 2017, nursing homes reported their staffing levels to CMS on the honor system. This self-reported staffing information was fed into the government's five-star rating system for nursing homes. Suspecting that the nursing-home industry may be inflating their staffing levels, CMS compared facility-reported staffing with payroll records from 2017 to 2018. The centers found that "more than half of the facilities analyzed met the expected staffing level less than 20 percent of the time."[67] Now that CMS is using payroll records, it is known that Medicare's five-star rating systems for nursing homes often exaggerated staffing level. Periods of low staffing were very rarely identified.[68]

More than fourteen thousand nursing homes submitted their payroll records for the CMS study. Seventy percent had lower staffing than their self-reporting had claimed. The average difference between self-reported and actual was 12 percent.[69]

Payroll records for the last quarter of 2017 showed that in a quarter of the facilities, there were no registered nurses at work for at least one day.[70] A study done by Harvard/Vanderbilt researchers in 2018 sounded another alarm bell. "In the weeks before and after the [CMS] survey week, mean staffing levels were higher than annual staffing level. Staffing levels increased before the survey week, reached a peak during the survey week, and then dropped following the survey."[71]

With payroll data providing more accurate information on staffing, CMS lowered ratings for some nursing homes that have gone for more than seven days with no registered nurse at all.[72]

Another flaw in the system, however, is that Medicare's five-star rating is created by comparing a nursing home to other nursing homes in the area. So even though a facility's staffing levels may now be known to be 12 percent lower than previously believed, their star rating could remain the same, depending on how other facilities in the area reported. Medicare's five-star ratings are done "on the curve."[73]

Weekends. David Grabowski, a member of the Harvard/Vanderbilt team that published their payroll staff hours study in *Health Affairs* in 2019, also sits on the Medicare Payment Advisory Commission. He said, "Staffing is the most important input into strong quality of care." The Harvard/Vanderbilt team found that nursing homes had "substantially lower" staffing on weekends compared to weekday business hours.[74]

Weekend staffing is always particularly difficult. Jay Vandemark, a middle-aged resident in a long-term care facility, summed up the atmosphere on weekends by saying, "It's almost like a ghost town." The chief operating officer of the facility where Vandemark lives gave a rationale for the lower staffing on weekends: employees were guaranteed every other weekend off, so it was difficult to get as many weekend staff as they would like. Medicare's examination of staff payroll records showed an average of "11 percent fewer nurses providing direct patient care on weekends and 8 percent fewer aides."

Dr. David Gifford, senior vice president of quality and regulatory affairs of the nursing-home industry trade group, American Health Care Association (AHCA), glossed over the lower staffing on weekends, despite the fact that residents still need to be dressed, toileted, and fed regardless of the day of the week. Said Gifford, "On weekends, there are fewer activities for residents and more family members around." The spouse of a woman resident in the same facility where Vandemark lives complained, "Weekends are terrible." He acknowledged that his own presence on weekends helped with his wife's care, but he wasn't buying Gifford's suggestion that family visits could substitute for adequate staffing on weekend. "What about all those other residents? They don't have people who come in."[75]

TIPS

- Remember that every minute of a CNA's time counts. Be polite and friendly, but don't engage them in prolonged chitchat because they have other patients to tend to.
- Visit nursinghome411.org for the latest info on staffing levels for every nursing home—in compliance with federal reporting requirements—and the top ten and bottom ten nursing homes in each state. Also available on this website are fact sheets on residents' rights from the Long Term Care Community Coalition.

CHAPTER 13
Coming to the End

As I drove toward the nursing home, I was struck with the realization that I was somewhat like a mythical creature, one who traveled freely between two worlds, the outside world and the nursing-home world. Then, within Mom's nursing-home world, I was also able to move between residents and staff.

In the everyday world, the world outside of the nursing home, my mythic self faded away, and I was quite ordinary. I was short, plump, gray-haired, and myopic. I dressed in comfortable clothes that are clean but never ironed. I didn't care if the color of my socks matched my slacks or picked up the color of my top. I spent more time brushing my teeth than fussing with my hair. And yet, the minute I strode into the nursing home, I felt myself to be the epitome of health and benevolence. I was a healthy woman, walking without a limp or walker. My hearing was excellent. My speech was both clear and loud enough to be easily heard and understood. I had enough money to buy anything I wanted to eat for lunch, could pay for a pair of eyeglasses, could drive my car anywhere I wanted to go, and had the wits to remember where my car keys were. And I always knew what day of the week it was!

In this journey with my mom, the focus was always on her. But just as a camera might capture the image of a butterfly you didn't even notice while you had been focusing the lens on a building, this saga of challenges I encountered in the nursing home wasn't only about the things I had learned in order to help her. It had also revealed facets of my personality and heart formerly invisible to me. Although childless, I found I *could* nurture someone. Embittered by years of emotional neglect from my mother, I found grace in forgiving her even though she hadn't asked for it. My heart was lighter than it had been in decades as we entered the final stretch of my mother's lifespan.

For supper, I brought her grated corn on the cob fresh from the farm. I mashed up a few slices of tomato from my sister's garden too. Mom ate with atypical gusto. I took her outside where the breeze was gentle and cool. I sang to her. As always, I stopped now and then for her to supply words for the songs. Tonight, she tried— even though she didn't succeed—to vary her pitch to fit in with the melody. It occurred to me that we were in totally uncharted seas. When the summer had begun, I'd merely hoped to help my mother die as peacefully and gracefully as possible. Could it be that all the stimulation and love and peanut butter pudding I had poured into her had helped her heal? I knew now that stroke patients could make gains.

"Mom, it has been just one year since you had your big stroke. Do you remember that?"

She looked at me incredulously. "A stroke?"

I talked her through the story, pausing often to give her a chance to process what I was saying and to respond if she wanted to. "You had a stroke when you were in your apartment alone. You were on the couch. Joe knocked on the door. 'Knock, knock, knock.' Then he knocked on your window. 'Knock, knock, knock.' You didn't answer, so he had to break through your window. He called 911. The ambulance came and took you to the hospital."

She looked like this was all news to her. I told her about the feeding tube and the months without food. She had no memory of any of this. Then I told her about removing the feeding tube and her hospitalization for pneumonia in February. Still no memory. The first recent memory she had was of the strawberry cheesecake for my birthday on April 28. She declared, "Charles didn't get a piece of that cake. I wanted Charles to have some of that cake." She was still distressed over this. I reassured her that Charles understood and was not upset.

So here we were. It was September 6, 2007, and her memory from September 2006 to April 2007 was gone. However, she still had some memory from April 28 to the present. There was no one who could or would help me make sense of this medically. It was just me,

Jenny, and my little mom out here, playing on a sandbar surrounded by an ocean of uncertainty. The waves of forgetfulness and death lapped over us as we patted our hands in the water, drawing shapes in the sand with our fingers. Occasionally, we looked up and waved at someone else. Sometimes, I sat her on my lap to keep her head above the waterline. So far, we had kept her from drowning in a sea of indifference.

"Mom," I asked. "What do you think the future will bring? What is going to happen now? What are your plans?"

This was new language for her. The future tense. I wondered if this was heady stuff for her and whether she recognized the significance of the tense shift.

I reflected on that day, thinking how being present to ask her these questions was a luxury probably enjoyed by no one else in her nursing home. I was acting as an amateur therapist, asking her to consider her hopes and dreams. I was willing to listen to what went on in her mind. The nursing home tried to keep residents clean, out of bed, dressed each day, fed, quiet, and protected from falls. Staff would say a few words, but no one reached out to the residents' hearts. I was, and still am, so grateful I was there for my mom to do that.

I had spent all summer with her, like a miner hammering away at a rock wall, seeking for one piece of ore, one precious stone, one word from her. And now that she was blossoming, I'd be taking that stimulus away from her because my sublet was over, and I was returning to Wisconsin. What would I do if Mom really did significantly improve? Would I move back here? Her father lived to be ninety-seven. She could too. That would be another seven years.

I had come here to help her die. Instead, I'd uncovered a completely new question: What would I do if my mother got better?

JOURNAL ENTRY 13-2

Mom was no longer in physical therapy or occupational therapy. Tom said my mom still received restorative therapy with him each day, but she was no longer able to hold any weight on her feet. She remained seated in her wheelchair and did leg lifts and moved her arms around. I was grateful for any break in the monotony of her days.

JOURNAL ENTRY 13-3

I came back in December and was surprised by how much the nursing home felt like home to me now. The lobby was all decorated for Christmas. It looked festive, and I liked it!

As usual, there was a flock of residents in the lounge, hoping for a little entertainment from the people passing by. I asked Little David how his mother was doing—they were both patients in the nursing home and shared a room. I kidded with Matt about the Phillies hat he wore. I stuck my head into the social worker's office to say hi to Mindy, but Mindy didn't work there anymore. Instead, I met her replacement, Brenda. I inwardly groaned. Another change in staff! Another important cog in the administrative wheel I would have to ingratiate myself to. Well, Christmas was a good time to do that!

Mom was not in the lounge, so I hurried as quickly as I could, without actually breaking into a run, to get down the hall, first to the dining room and then to Mom's room. By the time I reached her room, I was sweating and still wearing my coat. The nursing home kept the temperature really warm.

I couldn't restrain myself. I flung my coat onto her bed and jumped in next to her. "Mom! Mom, I'm back!"

Previous experience taught me not to expect my mother to be enthusiastic about my return. Once when I had come for a visit and hurried into her room full of good cheer and love, my mother said, "Oh, I hoped I would be dead before you came back." After that, I didn't expect anything emotional from her. I just contented myself with telling her how much I'd missed her. How much I loved her. And how cute, how adorable she was.

JOURNAL ENTRY 13-4

Mom's ninetieth birthday party was a huge success, if I do say so myself. Everyone came who said they would. Even Tom from the physical therapy staff stopped by for a few minutes. I guessed Mom had been able to communicate an invitation, as Jenny and I hadn't wanted to obligate him to come to the nursing home when he was off duty.

Jenny had found a crown with a soft headband decorated with faux amethysts for Mom. I draped a lavender boa around her neck. We brought in a boom box and played CDs of hymns, my mother's favorite music. We decorated the room with purple, pink, and white crepe paper. We continued the purple color scheme with plastic tablecloths, plates, and napkins. Her minister gave a speech.

We had requested no presents, but Charles brought her a bottle of maple syrup. She liked maple syrup on her morning Wheatina® cereal. Several people gave her bananas bedecked with ribbons and bows because, at the moment, bananas were her favorite thing to eat.

Later, when I looked at pictures of that day, I thought Mom looked happy. The only time I'd seen her happier was when her grandson visited. He was in the military, so he couldn't get away to visit her that day.

JOURNAL ENTRY 13-5

Christmas was rather anticlimactic for us after Mom's exciting birthday party. The party had also given us plenty of fodder for conversation with the staff.

My best Christmas present ever was Jenny announcing she and her husband were moving back to New Jersey early the next year. She would be only five miles from Pineville. I was thrilled for my mom and relieved for myself.

JOURNAL ENTRY 13-6

Jenny's move had taken place in March, and she was exemplary in taking care of Mom. Jenny visited the nursing home six days a week. Despite this frequent attendance, Mom's hearing aids continued to be as difficult to locate as ever. It was hit or miss whether Mom's glasses would be on her face when Jenny arrived. Jenny soaked Mom's hands in a basin of soapy water each day to get them truly clean; we had come to realize that the aides did not wash her hands other than during her weekly bathing.

Jenny also took on doing Mom's laundry. This was wonderful because Jenny folded and hung Mom's clothes so they weren't as wrinkled. Best of all, Jenny had figured out how to get the urine smell out of Mom's clothes, something the nursing-home laundry had failed to do. Jenny found that soaking clothes in Borax cleaner for half an hour before washing them would fix the problem.

I came back at this time because I was, to my own surprise, missing my mother. I also wanted to give Jenny a little vacation from going to the nursing home every day.

JOURNAL ENTRY 13-7

It was my birthday today, April 28. I had wondered if Mom would remember and try to do something again this year as she had done last year. But it was obvious she hadn't realized the date, so I didn't even mention it.

I showed her the pictures from Denmark again. She gave no indication that she had seen them earlier and dutifully repeated "Denmark" and "Copenhagen" after I said the words. I then decided to play a game with her. I first sang a song she knew well, "The Old Rugged Cross." As I sang, I tapped the rhythmic pattern on her arm. I did the same with "In the Garden." Then I told her I would silently sing a song in my head while tapping it onto her arm for her to guess.

I made sure to pick only those songs I knew she had been singing for at least eighty years: "Sweet Hour of Prayer," "Onward Christian Soldiers," and "Showers of Blessing." She loved it and she guessed each one correctly. Then she wanted a turn to tap on my arm. I had more trouble guessing than she did! This made her enjoy the game even more.

Before I knew it, it was time to bring her in for supper. I made sure they brought her egg salad, as I was still concerned about her weight—not that I had found the energy to ask the floor nurse how much she weighed— and whether she was getting enough protein. Charles had taken up the habit of bringing her extra bananas so she could have one whenever she wanted. But the floor nurse had taken me aside yesterday to tell me they didn't want Charles to do that anymore. Mom had one last banana left, so we shared it as a dessert after she had eaten all the egg salad she wanted.

Theoretically, an aide was to bring around a snack cart in the evening before bedtime. Rarely did this cart have fruit on it, and even more rarely did it have bananas. Mostly, what they offered were cookies and ice cream. Mom was still on pureed foods only, so she couldn't have the cookies and she was worried—I would not make this up—that the ice cream would make her fat. Why she would care about her weight when her hair looked like a troll doll's and several of her teeth were missing was beyond me. Once in a while, they had pudding cups, and she would take one. However, she couldn't peel back the foil lids on her own. If the aide didn't notice this and open it for her, I am sure the pudding remained uneaten.

JOURNAL ENTRY 13-8

When I had told Mom at lunch today that I'd be leaving for home the next day, she just said, "Oh," and turned her head away. I felt terrible to realize she was disappointed that I was leaving. I tried to reassure her that once I left, Jenny would be back to visiting her six days each week. I told her she wouldn't be alone. I would also still be checking up on her through calls to the nursing home and Jenny. Still, she refused to eat anything more.

Back in her room, I couldn't interest her in any of her picture books or my pictures of Denmark. She didn't want to play the tapping game either. She just wanted to go to bed, so I found Tom and asked him to settle her into bed for the night.

I went to the store and bought Mom some butterscotch pudding and bananas. I would have bought her anything on earth she was allowed to eat, but these were the only things I could think of that she would like. I was really sad about leaving and wondered why it had taken her until she was ninety to enjoy my company.

JOURNAL ENTRY 13-9

In July, my visit overlapped with my nephew's visit. He was strong enough to gently lift her out of her wheelchair and place her in the car without any difficulty. I told Mom we would drive her anywhere she wanted to go.

She didn't want to go far, just to where she thought her brother lived and to where her parents' farm used to be.

"What about Washington Crossing park?" I tried to tempt her. "New Hope? The Delaware River?"

No interest. But it didn't really matter because we weren't in the car for even ten minutes before she fretted about being away from the nursing home. She was afraid they wouldn't keep her bed open for her. She feared they would look for her and not find her. She was afraid she would be reported to the "guards" and punished. Her anxiety escalated so quickly that she was completely freaking out and seemed deaf to our reassurances. We turned the car around and took her back to the nursing home. Obviously, it now represented security to her.

JOURNAL ENTRY 13-10

I had very fond memories of Halloween at Pineville for the last two years, so I decided to time this visit to enjoy that holiday with my little mother. When I arrived, I noticed she was even more feeble than she had been in July, which I wouldn't have thought was possible.

Since her stroke, she never had enough strength to hold a normal fork or spoon in her hands to feed herself, but she could manage a plastic spoon for mashed potatoes or pudding. Now, it seemed she couldn't even manage this. The floor nurse told me if she couldn't feed herself, she would be placed at a table for those in advanced stages of dementia. I had seen how they fed her former roommate, Betty; they mixed her food with milk, then just tilted her head back and shoveled it in. I didn't know if they would do this to my mom since she still had compromised muscles in her throat for swallowing. But I preferred not to find out.

Getting Mom to handle a plastic spoon and feed herself was my number one priority for this visit. I explained to her, repeatedly, that if she gave up on using a spoon, she would be placed in the back room. I took her back there to show her what her future would be. That motivated her, and she focused her waning abilities on lifting a plastic spoon with a dab of food on it to her mouth.

JOURNAL ENTRY 13-11

Today was the Halloween parade. Mom wore her "costume"—the orange tee-shirt and orange striped socks—that she had worn the past two years. But our hearts weren't in the celebration this year and neither was Mom's. She was running out of energy and had little interest in anything. She wasn't charmed by the little children in their costumes. She didn't want to hand out candy. She didn't say "boo" to anyone.

END OF HER STORY

Since I had a sister visiting her every day, a husband in Denmark, and a job in Wisconsin, I only visited my mom a few times during her last year. I knew Jenny tried to keep Mom as comfortable and clean as possible. She also took care of Mom's paperwork. We had given up asking about Mom's weight or for a dentist to clean her teeth. Her clothes still fit, so we figured she was within the boundaries of where she should be.

The nursing home, despite all the precautions we had taken, lost her last hearing aid. We suspected they put it on the wrong patient and no one noticed. Mom never did adjust to her replacement glasses, so we didn't think she saw or heard much at all. Jenny said Mom didn't seem interested in having a conversation. Occasionally, she still asked for a banana, but that was about it.

In January 2010, we invited Jenny to visit us in Copenhagen. She was only willing to be gone for a week because she was so conscientious about Mom. After so many years, Mom's church visitors had dwindled to only her minister and the ever-faithful Charles.

Despite the freezing temperatures, we had a grand visit. We enjoyed a frigid excursion to Hamlet's Castle on the North Sea and a walk through Tivoli Gardens, still decked out for Christmas. After her flight home, Jenny called to let me know she had arrived safely back in New Jersey. She said she would visit Mom tomorrow because it was past visiting hours when she'd landed.

The next morning, while she was getting dressed, Jenny got a call from the nursing home. They said

Mom had passed away a few hours earlier. Our mother had developed shingles shortly before Jenny left for Copenhagen. The nurse thought the added stress of shingles pushed Mom across the line from the living to the deceased.

We knew Mom had literally been praying for death since her stroke in 2006. We also knew she honestly believed, with her whole heart and soul, that she would go straight to heaven to be with Jesus. I hope she is enjoying singing those old-time hymns as part of the heavenly chorus.

As I write this, it has been ten years since she died. I am still angry with the treatment we received from the nursing-home staff. Even more, I miss hearing her wobbly, little voice singing along with me, or feeling her little finger tapping out the rhythm of "Standing on the Promises."

MY REFLECTIONS

They say hindsight is twenty-twenty. I don't know if I am seeing twenty-twenty even now, several years after Mom's death; end-of-life issues, such as mental competency and stroke recovery, are complex in and of themselves. They are further complicated by a lifetime of emotional baggage and the pressures of finances and external time deadlines. But even if my hindsight isn't twenty-twenty yet, I believe I do see things *much* more clearly than I did while I was living through them. Here are some things I wish I'd had the sense to do differently.

I would have made much more of the summer between my mother's TIA in April 2006 and her big stroke on Labor Day in 2006. We had nearly three full months of Mom living in her apartment, between her temporary stay at Pineville for rehabilitation and her permanent stay at Pineville. During that summer interlude, she was lucid. She was still talking in complete sentences. It would have been a little inconvenient to help her walk with her walker to the car and drive her places, but it was still possible. At the time, Jenny and I thought she was on a gradual ascent in her mobility. We thought we could wait on some business matters until she had improved more.

We had no idea at the time that this interval was but a brief hiatus, a prelude to a more debilitating stroke. My mother's father had lived independently and quite happily until he fell and broke a rib when he was ninety-seven. My mother had enjoyed excellent health until her TIA when she was eighty-eight. Jenny and I both thought Mom would have a few more years of relatively good health.

Statistically, people who suffer a TIA are at high risk for another stroke soon thereafter. My mother's doctor never communicated this to us. Had I known, I think I would have tried to accomplish the following things during the interval we had: sign over my mother's car to my sister, take my mother to the bank and have her put my sister on her bank account as a cosignor, take her to the optometrist for an exam and new glasses, and have a serious discussion with her about those end-of-life decisions on an advance medical directive. Had Jenny and I known that Mom was so opposed to extreme measures to keep her alive, we may not have called the neighbor to check on her on Labor Day. We definitely would not have consented to the stomach feeding tube.

I would like to think I would have made more of this interval in another way, by spending the summer of 2006 with her. I would have encouraged her to physically improve as much as possible and maybe even tried to build up her upper-body strength. I'm not positive I would have done this because my job was also important to me. I'd like to think I would have chosen to spend the entire summer of 2006 with her anyway, encouraging her to walk, hydrate herself, and lift light weights. I believe if Mom had been stronger when the big stroke hit, she would have recovered more afterward. This is just my hypothesis; I don't know for sure.

I would have insisted we find a different doctor for my mother—or, at least, I would have tried to insist; she could be very stubborn. After the TIA, my mother was still in good enough physical shape that we could have taken her doctor shopping. But after the first TIA, we figured Mom would be back to living independently soon and therefore, it wasn't really our business to interfere in her selection of a doctor. Dr. Adams had been her doctor and Aunt Molly's doctor for several years, which had caused Jenny and me to think that our mother and aunt were satisfied with his service. Then, after the big stroke, when we thought she was dying very soon, there wasn't much point in changing doctors.

Would I have moved Mom to Wisconsin during the summer of 2006 had I known she would be going into a nursing home permanently come September? I'd like to say the answer is "yes." It would have made my life easier in some ways. I could have visited her every day without quitting my job. And I believe, although I have no proof, that the nursing homes in my area are better than those in Mom's area. Plus, in Wisconsin, I was better connected socially to people in the health field with whom I could have consulted regarding my mother. It had been thirty-five years since I'd lived in New Jersey, so I had no social contacts with medical professionals there.

But even in my nearly perfect hindsight, I have to remember that my mother lived all but three years of her life within ten miles of her birthplace, and her friends at church had always meant more to her than her family. As long as Mom was mentally competent, she would never have consented to a move to Wisconsin. So in the final analysis, the answer is no, I would not have moved her to Wisconsin.

The most important thing I wish I had realized sooner was not to expect the medical professionals to *ever* tell us anything. I wish I had known to get busy and do research on my own, immediately. We waited too long for the professionals to tell us things, and in most cases, they never did.

I wish I had more deeply researched stroke recovery, aphasia, and music therapy online. I could have been more effective during the summer of 2007 in helping my mom talk again. I should have researched sooner the rights of nursing-home residents and their caregivers. I wish I had questioned the formula they were giving Mom when she had the feeding tube; I learned later from a registered dietitian that there are several types of these formulas. A high-protein variety would have better promoted healing of her bedsores.

I still wish someone would tell me the best way to ask for anything from a staff person at the nursing home. That remains a mystery. But as I have included advice and tips for people with loved ones residing in long-term care facilities throughout this book, I feel empowered to share some tips for nursing-home staff as they deal with us.

SUGGESTIONS TO THE STAFF

- Wear your name tags so we can see your name. Why not put your name on *both* sides of your name tag?
- Give us a checklist that includes important topics such as "dentist," "vision," and "bathing" with simple descriptions of your services and how to obtain them. For example, how do we get our loved one on the list to see the dentist? How

much will a visit cost and to whom do we give the check? Also, what services are possible?

- Please be more transparent with us. If, for example, your facility has decided that staff will never groom fingernails, please tell us so we can figure out an alternative strategy to clean, cut, and file nails.
- Start off by assuming that we are honest and decent people. If we prove you wrong, then of course you can adjust your dealings with us accordingly.
- Have aides spend two to three hours in sensitivity training to learn how to see things from the patient's perspective. Stuff their ears with cotton to make hearing a little difficult, wear oversize gloves to simulate lack of motor coordination, and put goggles smeared with Vaseline on their eyes to provide a taste of obstructed vision. It is the only way I can think of to make aides more sensitive to not losing glasses and hearing aids and to get them to open yogurt cups.
- Keep a file with blank copies of important paperwork, such as advance medical directives and do-not-hospitalize forms, in the nursing home office. One sheet of paper should summarize what's needed, with bullet-point lists of the number of witnesses needed, whether a notary is required, and who should receive and file the completed and signed form within the nursing home.

- Follow-up with nursing-home staff regarding weight checks.
- Create a laminated card with a few basic pictures (or words) on it so a patient can point to the words such as "pain," "cold," "water," and so on. Many aides do not speak English clearly, and many patients have garbled speech (or no speech at all). This card would save many misunderstandings and be a good starting point to improve communication.

The Need for Reform

The year 2020 will forever be known as "the year of COVID-19." This is a novel virus, which means it has never been identified in humans, and we are required to learn about it as we live (and die) through it. At the beginning, we were told there were three hard and fast symptoms: fever, dry cough, and shortness of breath. Those without these three symptoms could rest assured that they did not have COVID-19. Stores sold out of their thermometers within a few days. The original short list of these three symptoms defining COVID-19 has now given way to a new list of possible symptoms that is still expanding: chills, fatigue, muscle aches, headache, loss of taste, loss of smell, sore throat, runny nose, nausea, vomiting, and diarrhea. We were told the only way to find out if you had it was to be tested, but for many long weeks, there were precious few tests to be had, and those that did exist seemed directed to the rich and famous such as Tom Hanks, George Stephanopolous, and professional basketball players. The rest of us were told to just stay home if we didn't feel sick enough to be admitted to the hospital.

What about those who had no choice but to stay put in their nursing homes and other long-term care facilities? We will never know the true number of long-term care facility residents who had COVID-19 and how many of them died. According to a June 2020 article in *USA Today*, more than 9,600 long-term care facilities in the United States have had at least one case. Over 208,000 residents and staff have tested positive.[76]

The spread of COVID-19 has given media attention to nursing homes, particularly their standard of care for infectious illnesses. In 2016, the Obama administration mandated planning by nursing-homes for hazards and emergencies such as Ebola. Shortly after Trump's election, the American Health Care Association—AHCA is the largest nursing home lobby in the United States—wrote to the president and expressed their hope that his administration would reduce the "extremely burdensome" rules that governed their ultimate profit margin.[77]

The Trump administration affirmed that nursing homes did need to have specific plans to handle unfamiliar and contagious diseases. Despite this clarification of the rule, inspectors found violations in 6,599 nursing homes between November 2017, when the rule took effect, and March 2020. This meant 43 percent of nursing homes in the United States had not been adequately prepared for an emergency outbreak such as COVID-19.[78]

According to a 2018 report of the United States Senate Committee on Finance not only were many nursing homes unprepared for a disease pandemic, they were even unprepared for more common disasters such as hurricanes. Nursing homes were supposed to write emergency plans and train employees on implementation of these plans. Too often, inspectors found there had been no training of employees and no rehearsals in mock drills.[79]

The Health and Human Services Office of Inspector General (OIG) concluded in 2019 that inspectors in five states failed to police the implementation of the emergency preparedness rule for nursing homes. Those states were California, New York, Florida, Texas, and Missouri.[80] In California, 95 percent of nursing homes dealing with COVID-19 had been cited for deficiencies in their emergency plans for infectious diseases.[81]

We will probably never know with certainty how many long-term care residents died from coronavirus. This is partially due to lack of testing in the early months and partially due to underreporting. As of May 22, 2020, seven states have not reported their COVID-19 statistics for long-term care facilities at all.[82] Further, the Trump administration has said it will not require nursing homes to provide data on confirmed COVID-19 cases and deaths that occurred prior to May 6, 2020.[83] What we do know, or think we know, has been pieced together by data collected by news outlets and individual states. A May 22, 2020, estimate by the Foundation for Research on Equal Opportunity is that 42 percent were in nursing homes and assisted-living facilities.[84] In some states, that percentage is much higher—70 percent of COVID-19 deaths in Ohio and 69 percent in Pennsylvania.[85] A *Washington Post* article in June estimated thirty-two thousand residents and six hundred employees of nursing homes died due to COVID-19 nationally.[86]

These estimates are bound to change as more hard data trickles in. What we do know is that these facilities are especially prone to infectious outbreaks, not only due to the age and underlying conditions of their residents and lack of emergency preparedness plans by administrators but also because many of the staff go from nursing home to nursing home, spreading the virus as they travel via X-ray technicians, hospice workers, phlebotomists and more. Even within the same nursing home, inspectors found that 33 percent of nurses and aides did not wash their hands properly, and 25 percent used personal protection equipment (PPE) incorrectly even once the pandemic was underway.[87] The threat of fines was not enough to change this behavior. "The fines are so small that they don't really have an impact on the nursing home," said Charlene Harrington, a professor of Nursing and Sociology at the University of California, San Francisco.[88]

The first easy fix suggested to halt the spread of the virus was checking temperatures of visitors and staff before they entered a facility. This obviously was not enough as we later learned that many with the virus fail to show a fever.[89] Up to 80 percent of those testing positive report only mild symptoms, and 18 percent are completely asymptomatic.[90] So simply screening with a thermometer will not find all carriers of the infection!

Lack of sufficient PPE exacerbated the spread of the virus. Many nursing homes lacked any surgical masks at all, and many hundreds said their supply of masks would last less than a week. More than eight hundred reported they were a week away from running out of hand sanitizer. The AHCA lobbied the federal government to help nursing homes obtain face masks, gloves, disposable gowns, and so on. The Department of Health and Human Services did allocate $4.9 billion for that purpose, but it wasn't until May 21 and even then, the AHCA said this was not nearly enough.[91] At that point, worldwide supplies of PPE were extremely low. Money was allocated, but there were little to no PPE supplies available for purchase. It was a case of too little, too late. In May, Federal Emergency Management Agency (FEMA) announced that each nursing home would receive two shipments—each with a one-week supply of PPE—by July 4.[92] Also critical was the lack of tests, which meant nursing homes didn't know which residents and staff members needed to be isolated.[93]

The AHCA asked Congress for an additional $10 billion dollars to pay for additional staff and bonuses for hazard pay and to make up for their financial losses caused by having to close their facilities to new residents.[94]

Shortage of staff severely impacted nursing homes trying to stop the spread of COVID-19. More than 2,200 facilities said they lacked enough aides.[95] Charlene

Harrington directly connects the severity of COVID-19 in nursing homes to shortages in staffing.[96]

If I had the power to change the long-term care system, I would focus first on three areas: staffing, enforcement of already-existing regulations, and an end to illegal evictions of residents. With direct lines already drawn between insufficient staff and nursing-home COVID-19 rates, need for additional staffing should take top priority in every state.

Staffing. Even without a pandemic pushing conditions to an extreme, many studies have found a high correlation between low staffing and low quality of care, which only stands to reason. This may seem obvious, but experts estimate that only 5 percent of nursing homes are adequately staffed.[97]

The current federal regulations on staffing are not very detailed; a minimum of one RN must be on the premises eight consecutive hours, seven days each week, and an LPN must be on the premises twenty-four hours each and every day. But there is no federal mandate covering CNA staffing, only that it must be "sufficient" to meet the needs of the residents.[98]

In my opinion, the need for higher staffing should start with increasing the number of CNAs. Who does the call bell summon in a nursing home? In the vast majority of cases, it is a CNA who will arrive. They are the ones who give the bulk of direct patient care such as toileting, dressing, bathing, brushing teeth, repositioning to avoid bedsores, finding personal items such as hearing aids, and feeding. As I and others have observed, these things are not always getting done in our nursing homes.

Residents in understaffed facilities are at a higher risk of malnutrition, weight loss, bedsores, falls, and infections.[99] Over 150 studies have been undertaken on the relationship between staffing and quality of care. The strongest correlation is between RN hours and outcomes. But total staffing levels (including CNAs) are also positively correlated to quality.[100]

Not only does understaffing provide quality of life issues, but it is "one of the underlying causes of elder abuse and neglect in nursing homes."[101] Again, this would seem to be a logical correlation because overworked staff are more likely to make mistakes or fail to notice warning signs that something is amiss with a resident.

Further, highly stressed staff are more likely to commit elder abuse deliberately or because their difficult and frustrating work environment led to harmful but unintentional abuse.[102] Elder abuse in long-term care institutions is high. The World Health Organization says two out of three staff have reported they have committed abuse on the residents in their care in the past year.[103]

A particularly cruel twist on staff abusing nursing-home residents occurred in Danby House, an elder-care and assisted-living facility in Winston-Salem, North Carolina, in 2019. Three staff members filmed two residents in a dementia unit as staff urged residents to physically fight with each other. One of the residents was seventy years old and the other was seventy-three. One of them was filmed shouting for help, but the staff members ignored these pleas. Acting on a tip, the Winston-Salem police department investigated. The three staff members were arrested and charged with misdemeanors. NC Department of Health and Human Services suspended the facility from taking new patients and outlined multiple violations related to patient care.[104]

The Health and Human Services Office of Inspector General (OIG) reported in 2014 that 33 percent of nursing-home residents experienced adverse events resulting in harm or death during their first thirty-five days of admission to a long-term care facility from a hospital. The same study found 50 percent of those adverse events related to substandard treatment, inadequate monitoring, or delays in treatment. The estimated cost to Medicare of $2.8 billion is all attributable to understaffing.[105]

With publicly documented cases of elder abuse in long-term care facilities, some families have turned to placing nanny cams—spy cameras—in the rooms of their loved ones. Steve Piskor filed four complaints with the nursing home about his concerns for his mother, Esther, without any action from the nursing-home administration. So he placed a camera in his mother's room, but the administrators told staff they could cover the camera lens with a towel. After seeing red welts on his mother's face, Piskor then hid a camera but put a sign up in the room stating there was a hidden camera. Despite the warning sign, Piskor obtained footage of aides slamming his mother into her wheelchair, pushing her face against the wall, and punching her in the face. The nursing home did not take Piskor's concerns seriously and told him he was "taking things out of context" and made him out to be a "bad guy" for complaining. The Ohio Department of Health has since cited the Elisabeth Severance Prentiss Center for Skilled Nursing and Rehabilitation for failing to prevent the abuse. Two of the nurses' aides were fired, and a third was disciplined. Esther died in 2018, but her son is working to convince the Ohio General Assembly to enact a law that will give families the right to place video cameras in nursing-home rooms.[106]

Esther Piskor's case is not unique. Camera footage has shown abuses at other nursing homes. For example, staff members shoving a latex glove into a resident's mouth, or a staff member sexually abusing a disabled resident. As of August 2019, the following states permit private cameras in nursing homes: Illinois, Kansas, Louisiana, Maryland, New Mexico, Oklahoma, Texas, Utah, Vermont, and Washington. Fifteen more states are considering the issue.[107]

Another trend in nursing-home populations that has increased the burden on staffing is an increase in residents who are mentally ill. There were over five hundred thousand such residents in 2005, and that excludes those with dementia. Persons with mental illness admitted to nursing homes tend to be quite a bit younger than the general nursing-home population—54 percent of them are between the ages of eighteen and sixty-four.[108] Whether it is ideal, or even desirable, for the mentally ill to be placed in nursing homes, the fact remains that until the dearth of other residential facilities is ameliorated, this will continue to be another factor demanding more of the nursing-home staff's time and resources. The overall physical health and strength of these relatively younger nursing-home residents can make them even more challenging when their illnesses make them violent or chaotic.

By and large, nursing homes are understaffed, and that understaffing leads to negligence, suffering, and sometimes, even abuse. There is no consensus, however, as to what constitutes a sufficient amount of CNA time per day for a resident—keeping in mind that if mentally ill patients or patients with complex medical conditions are in the mix, adjustments will need to be made to increase staffing levels to compensate. A glimpse of the workloads many CNAs struggle under is provided by an informal online poll: the average CNA has sixteen residents, and in Georgia, the maximum can be thirty residents.[109]

In the absence of any clear guidance by CMS Centers for Medicare and Medicaid, some states have adopted their own approaches to improving CNA staffing. It may be tempting to estimate the number of hours needed for each resident and mandate staff accordingly. Some states have gone this route, but this could be difficult to monitor for compliance; setting ratios of resident caseload per CNA would probably be easier to monitor. Some states have tried to tackle this issue by mandating maximum CNA-to-resident ratios. For example, legislation was introduced in the New Jersey General Assembly in January 2018—NJ Assembly bill 382—calling for each day-shift CNA to have no more than eight residents to care for. Evening-shift CNAs would have a maximum of ten residents, and on the night shift, sixteen would be the maximum.[110] Unfortunately, this bill did not make it through the New Jersey Senate.

As I suggested in Chapter 12, a good exercise is to do the math. Obviously, thirty minutes per day of direct patient care is not enough. Even in the absence of a state-mandated ratio, there is no rule against a nursing home deciding to employ more CNAs. After all, their labor costs are relatively low. The average hourly rate for CNAs in nursing homes in 2020 was thirteen to fourteen dollars per hour.[111] So why aren't more long-term care facilities doing this?

Some argue that it is hard to find and retain CNAs in sufficient numbers. Right now, when a starting employee at a fast-food restaurant can expect ten to twelve dollars an hour—sometimes with benefits such as tuition assistance—without undue risk to his back from transferring heavy residents out of bed and into a shower or exposure to deadly infections (MRSA), why would a young person choose a nursing-home position over one at a burger joint? In 2018, it was estimated that 48 percent of residential aides were considered low income for the purposes of eligibility for various forms of public assistance. It can't be argued that all of these workers are immigrants and, therefore, happy to work for low wages—79 percent of CNAs were born in the United States.[112] The hourly rate for CNAs needs to be increased to a living wage, depending on the geographic location.

Increasing the number of CNA hours and hourly wage levels would cut into profit margins. This is a critical factor when you consider that two-thirds of nursing homes are investor owned.[113] They are providing this service for a profit. There is nothing wrong with making a profit, and I am not suggesting that all nursing homes should be nonprofits. However, low staffing is often linked to a facility being for-profit. For-profit nursing homes and chains generally operate with fewer staff and provide lower quality of care as compared to nonprofit facilities. "Facilities with the highest profit margins have been found to have the poorest quality."[114]

An article by the Center for Medicare Advocacy asks if it makes a difference whether a long-term care facility is a for-profit corporate facility or a nonprofit. Their answer is a resounding yes despite the fact that some for-profits do give good care and some nonprofits provide poor care. They base their conclusion on eighty-two studies, comparing quality between the two types of ownership. Nearly all of the studies found higher quality, higher staffing, and few pressure sores in nonprofit facilities. They also had a lower use of restraints and fewer deficiencies found on government inspections. Based on these eighty-two studies, they postulated that if all US nursing homes were nonprofit, "seven thousand residents with pressure sores would not have them and residents would receive five hundred thousand more hours of nursing care each day."[115]

A different study approached the issue of for-profit and nonprofit ownership by looking at 1,149 nursing-home patients aged sixty and older who were seen at five hospitals in the Chicago area between 2007 and 2011. This research looked at twenty-four clinical signs, including constipation, dehydration, pressure ulcers, and broken catheter tubes. The researchers concluded there were more incidences of these clinical signs of neglect—including severe dehydration of patients with feeding tubes and poorly managed medications—among residents of the for-profit facilities.[116]

Yes, nursing homes are a profit-driven industry. The eighty-nine thousand long-term care facilities in the United States generated $250 billion annual revenue in 2019.[117] Capping nursing home profits is not the answer. We need to let our government know that the public would like to see those profits made without compromising the quality of care in nursing homes or reducing hardworking CNAs to dependence on some form of public assistance to get by. Let our states set reasonable staff ratios and then enforce them.

Enforcement of Regulations. Just writing and passing a law or regulation is only the first step in ensuring that good intentions translate into real-world practice. Nursing homes have grown used to breaking the rules already in place with little or no consequences. Current regulations governing quality of care and patients' rights as well as (hopefully) new rules for adequate staffing will need inspections and meaningful sanctions. Further, these inspections need to be transparent and the information gleaned made available to the public so consumers of nursing-home care can be knowledgeable in their choice of a facility.

In an odd twist, the federal government (through CMS) sets minimum nursing-home standards but leaves the states to inspect and determine if these standards are met. In order to receive Medicare and Medicaid payments, a facility must meet the standards in 42 C.F.R. Part 483 Subpart B. States certify facilities' compliance with CMS standards through annual inspections. If necessary, the states also have a responsibility to follow up on complaints and reports of misconduct, negligence, and adverse incidents.[118]

What sanctions does the government currently have in its enforcement arsenal? For violations of CMS regulations, Medicare may issue a fine, require in-service training to remedy a deficit in care, deny payment to the nursing home, assign a temporary manager, or install a state monitor.

But in reality, "Nursing homes are seldom terminated from a Medicare/Medicaid program as a result of violations. Within the US regulatory environment, the enforcement of current staffing requirements has been weak."[119] It has been suggested that putting holds on new-patient admissions of residents until deficiencies are remedied would be a good way to ensure timely compliance.

In October 2016, the CMS issued "Medicare & Medicaid Programs; Requirements for Long-Term Care Facilties: Regulatory Provisions to Promote Efficiency and Transparency" This rule strengthened requirements in areas such as infection control and quality improvement.[120] It also imposed requirements aimed at moving care to be more person-centered. The AHCA characterized the 2016 rule as "unnecessary, overly burdensome, and [getting] in the way of resident care." The AHCA has requested a shift in nursing-home oversight from government enforcement of regulations to a collaborative approach in which providers and regulators work together. From the AHCA point of view, the use of civil monetary penalties has been "out of control" and takes resources away from resident care. Again, resident advocates have expressed a different view, with one prominent advocate countering that penalties were finally at a level "that gets the industry's attention and isn't just viewed as the cost of doing business."[121]

What are the roadblocks to enforcing stronger regulations? There is a difference in opinion and philosophy in political factions between advocates for residents and industry managers and investors. The crux of the matter is that long-term care facilities "chafe under a system they find inflexible, ineffective, and overly prescriptive," while resident advocates believe widespread and egregious violations of standards for quality care demand robust, regulatory protocols. The scales should be tipped in favor of the protection of frail, elderly residents when changes in the current regulatory system are considered.[122]

The nursing-home industry has deep pockets, however, to sway legislators at both the federal and state levels as they write and pass new regulations. Between 2006 and 2009, the health sector contributed $1.7 billion in lobbying the US Congress and federal agencies. In Kentucky alone, the nursing-home industry gave $1.8 million to Kentucky politicians over a ten-year period.[123] The revolving door between politicians who leave office and become lobbyists and government hires of health industry managers helps explain why public officials and industry owners hold similar views that are heavily in favor of industry self-regulation rather than governmental regulatory approaches.

And who is there to counterbalance the billions of dollars paid to sway politicians to the industry's point of view? Consumer advocacy groups, which are primarily low-budget, volunteer-based entities. "Although there has been a large growth in old-age interest groups in the US, the effectiveness of their advocacy has been questionable and very few of these advocacy groups focus on nursing home issues."[124]

The current political climate favors a trend toward deregulation in all aspects of life in the United States. Yet it should be noted that plenty of for-profit businesses are burdened by a great deal of regulation. A case in point is the restaurant industry. Annually, this industry has revenues of $863 billion and employs over fifteen million workers in more than one million locations.[125] Yet it is precisely because of the regulatory burden of inspections that the public feels confident that patronizing these businesses will not put their health in jeopardy. If it were not for government inspections and sanctions, it is unlikely the restaurant industry would be as popular as it is. Why shouldn't we extend the same protection of government regulation to our fragile citizens in long-term care facilities?

Exit strategy. A 2017 headline in *Forbes* screamed, "Outrageous! Nursing Home Illegally Dumps Elderly Resident They Don't Want" and chronicled the experience of one elderly couple—the wife was evicted, but the husband was allowed to stay.[126] This is far from an isolated instance, and I am grateful it did not occur to my mother. But this practice is so heinous that I feel it needs to be included here.

The number one reported problem concerning nursing homes is that of discharging or evicting residents. Nursing-home ombudsmen received 10,610 such complaints nationally in 2017. CMS estimates as many as one-third of all residents in long-term care facilities are discharged involuntarily.[127] In California, improper-eviction complaints rose 70 percent over five years ending in 2017. In Illinois, involuntary-discharge complaints doubled from 2011 to 2017.[128]

Under federal law, a nursing home cannot transfer or discharge a resident from the nursing home where they are living unless:

A. The resident's needs cannot be met by the facility.

B. The resident's health has improved enough so they no longer need the services provided by the facility.

C. The safety of staff or other residents is endangered by the resident.

D. The health of other individuals in the facility is endangered.

E. The resident has failed, after reasonable and appropriate notice, to pay for their stay in the facility. Nonpayment would include situations where the resident, or his representative, has failed to submit the paperwork for Medicaid.

F. The facility ceases to operate.[129]

Federal law says a nursing home must give a thirty-day notice in writing before they evict someone.

If a resident feels they have been discharged improperly, they may appeal the discharge,[130] and the facility cannot evict them while their appeal is pending unless the failure to discharge the resident would endanger the health or safety of the resident or other individuals in the facility.[131]

The exception to the rule about not discharging a resident for lack of payment can occur if the nursing home does not accept Medicaid residents.[132] Those facilities that do not accept Medicaid can discharge for lack of payment. The other way a nursing home can get rid of a resident is to transfer them to a hospital and then refuse to readmit them on discharge from the hospital. The rules about how long a nursing home must hold a resident's bed for them while they are in the hospital vary by state. But even if the nursing home discharges a resident to a hospital and does not readmit them, they are still required to provide a care plan for the resident and make sure they have a safe place to go.[133]

The notice given to a resident of a facility's intention to discharge them must be in writing. Federal regulations require a facility to record the following: (1) the reason for the discharge and (2) any specific unmet needs and efforts made by the facility to meet those needs if the cause for eviction is the facility's inability to meet the resident's needs. If the reason for discharge is that the resident has improved enough to not need the services of the facility, then the resident's physician must give documentation of this status.[134]

Further, the facility must provide sufficient preparation and orientation to residents before they are evicted or transferred to ensure a safe and orderly transfer.

Generally, the reason a nursing home would want to evict a resident reflects the income the resident brings to the facility. Looking at the reimbursement rates in California can serve to illustrate the revenue difference between Medicare and Medicaid residents. According to the California Association of Health Facilities, while Medicare may reimburse more than $1,000 per day, those payments only continue for up to twenty days. The average California Medicaid reimbursement is $219 per day. It is illegal to evict residents based on the amount of payment, but it happens all too often. It is easy to see the temptation there would be to trade in a "low-rent" occupant of a bed for one who paid five times that rate.[135]

One example is Ronald Anderson, who was fifty-one and recuperating in a nursing home after a partial foot amputation. The staff woke him one night and loaded him into a van. They dumped him in his wheelchair in downtown Los Angeles, in an area with a large homeless population. The staff left him there without his insulin or testing kit. He now lives in a homeless shelter. The nursing home later paid $450,000 to settle the case. The money went to fines, better training of nursing-home staff, and finding temporary housing for other former residents made homeless.[136]

Ronald Anderson is not an isolated case. The director of the Union Rescue Mission in Los Angeles said resident dumping by nursing homes has become so common, they have set up a surveillance camera outside to try to catch the people doing the dumping of nursing-home residents.[137]

Anita Willis is another example. She was in a nursing home in California, recovering from a stroke. Medicaid told the nursing home it would no longer continue to pay for Willis's stay, and the nursing home gave Willis less than twenty-four hours to leave or pay $336 per day to continue. She couldn't afford to pay, so she left the nursing home and then bounced between budget motels, friends' couches, hospital ERs, and the occasional night in a car. Willis also suffered from an aneurysm, an ulcer, muscle weakness, gastritis, anemia, heart disease, and kidney disease. She was one of 1,504 such evictions in California in 2016. With the help of California Advocates for Nursing Home Reform, Willis appealed her eviction. During the hearing, she said she felt sick, was taken to the hospital by an ambulance, and was admitted for a torn aorta and bleeding ulcer. Willis ultimately lost her appeal. The judge ruled she had left "voluntarily" because she refused the "opportunity" to pay for her care herself even though payment for three days at the nursing home would have exhausted her disability income.[138]

Sometimes, nursing homes will pay for one or two nights for a resident to stay at a budget motel to get them out of their facility. Then they abandon them. Another facility discharged a resident to a storage unit on a hot summer day.[139]

In 2016, CMS strengthened requirements for nursing homes seeking to rid themselves of low-paying residents through discharges and transfers. One of the new requirements is that a resident can't be evicted for nonpayment if they are either applying for Medicaid or appealing a Medicaid denial. But other measures to end evictions have been modest: a $784,630 program to train nursing-home staff on proper procedures for a discharge in California and $84,000 for a smaller program in Montana. Otherwise, the CMS is simply encouraging states to create and pay for initiatives that would deal with facility-initiated discharges.[140]

It would be helpful for nursing homes to do a thorough job of evaluating a prospective resident before admitting them. Most prospective residents with needs the facility cannot meet would be weeded out this way, leading to fewer evictions in the future. According to the Omnibus Budget Reconciliation Act of 1987, people applying for admission to a nursing home must go through a preadmission screening to identify those with mental illness. Further, they are "prohibited from admitting any individual with a serious mental illness unless the State Mental Health Authority determines that the nursing home's level of care is required for that individual."[63] In reality, the OIG found that fewer than half of the nursing-home residents with a major mental illness were properly evaluated in the preadmission screening.[141]

Advocacy groups say the federal government could do a better job of enforcing the rules against evictions by making fines for such actions more substantial. It used to be that facilities were fined for each day of a violation. Since July 2017, they have been fined only once per violation. This means a nursing home that evicts a resident only gets one fine instead of a fine for each day the resident is denied access to a bed. According to Dr. David Gifford, fines of US nursing homes in the first eighteen months after the change in guidelines were about $47 million less as compared to the previous eighteen-month period. Gifford told NBC News the changes were not about saving the industry money but were meant to ensure consistent standards.[142]

Should it be the responsibility of long-term care facilities to ensure the safe and orderly transfer of a resident to a different location? Deborah Pacyna, spokeswoman for the California Association of Health Facilities, a trade organization that represents nursing homes, thinks not. She questions why nursing homes should be responsible for "providing a safety net for the indigent and homeless."[143] Whether or not her organization is happy with the concept, the fact is that this is current federal law.

As a society, we need to send a clear message to nursing homes that we find the practice of dumping our fragile elderly out of nursing homes to be vile and reprehensible. We need state inspectors and ombudsmen to enforce the law prohibiting this action. It is time to put these places out of business.

TIPS

- A nursing home must send written notice to the resident, the resident's designated representative, and the state's long-term care ombudsman thirty days before the planned discharge date. If the resident wants to remain in that facility, they can appeal the discharge and demand a hearing. The facility cannot discharge the resident while the appeal is pending, nor can they force someone to leave if they have applied for Medicaid and are waiting for a response.[144]

- Nursing-home reform is urgently needed. Appeals to an owner of a nursing home, or homes, are likely to fall on deaf ears. Such reform will only come when members of the public demand it from their political representatives at state and federal levels. Join organizations such as the National Consumer Voice for Quality Long-Term Care, (https://theconsumervoice.org/), Massachusetts Advocates for Nursing Home Reform (https://www.manhr.org/), and Friends of Residents in Long Term Care (https://forltc.org/).
- The National Consumer Voice for Long-Term Care includes advocacy-skills training on its website.
- Any bruises, cuts, or bedsores on your loved one should be documented and photographed if you suspect there may be abuse by the nursing-home staff.
- Placement of video cameras in residents' rooms should not occur without consultation of state guidelines. Be aware that if you place a hidden camera in a nursing home, some states permit the nursing home to remove the resident and bring charges against you.

Conclusion

This is America, and it would be anathema to suggest we do away with for-profit nursing homes. But it is crucial we balance this drive for profit with governmental oversight, inspections, and sanctions to ensure the well-being of our frail elderly. We need to have nursing-home staff who are properly trained, compensated, and valued as a vital component of our long-term care system.

We need to do whatever is necessary to stop the practice of dumping our frail elderly on the street, in homeless shelters, and on sidewalks. If the owners of nursing homes value profit over the dignity of human life to the extent they will direct employees to undertake this action, then, collectively, we need to make them understand, by whatever methods that would be effective, that this is unacceptable.

Acknowledgments

I thank my friend, Liz Hill, for patiently listening to me while I lived through those nursing home years with my mother and wrote this book. I am grateful to my boss in Eau Claire, Wisconsin for those months and years when she granted me the flexibility to re-arrange my work schedule to visit my mother.

The early readers of this book are stalwart friends who contributed their honest and thoughtful comments: Kenn Amdahl, Carol Bjorlie, Dea Brayden, Diane Emon, Linda Hauschild, Nancy Imhof, Carolyn Keating, and Jean Teuch. I appreciate your feedback more than you can know.

I owe an immense debt of gratitude to those who let me interview them for this book. You shall remain anonymous, however, as that was my promise to you before we began our interviews.

Finally, I thank my sister without whom I would not have survived all the obstacles and annoyances thrown at us by the nursing home. You are the best! I am so grateful you are my sister.

Endnotes

Introduction

1 Atul Gawande, *Being Mortal* (New York: Picador of Henry Holt and Company, 2014).

2 Elaine Howley, "Nursing Home Facts and Statistics," *U.S. News and World Report*, October 11, 2019; Rebecca Laes-Kushner, "Skilled Nursing Facilities: Too Many Beds" (PDF), online supplement of *University of Massachusetts Medical School*, (Massachusetts: Commonwealth Medicine Publications, 2018), https://escholarship. umassmed.edu/cgi/viewcontent.cgi?article=1201&context=commed_pubs; James Hill, "Consider Nursing Home Optometry as Practice Option," *Optometry Times*, April 18, 2017.

3 Pierre Amarenco et al., "One-Year Risk of Stroke after Transient Ischemic Attack or Minor Stroke," *New England Journal of Medicine* 374, no. 16 (April 2016): 1533–1542, https://doi.org/10.1056/NEJMoa1412981.

4 Anna Medaris Miller, "7 Red Flags to Watch for when Choosing a Nursing Home," *U.S. News and World Report*, March 5, 2015.

5 "Left Untreated, Bedsores Can be Lethal," *South Florida Sun Sentinel*, May 19, 2014.

6 Carol Bradley Bursack, "What Every Caregiver Should Know About Bed Sores," AgingCare, May 19, 2020, https://www.agingcare.com/articles/what-caregivers-need-to-know-about-bed- sores-203147.htm.

7 Bursack, "About Bed Sores."

8 Sarah Lyon, "What to do if your Loved One Develops a Bedsore in a Nursing Home," *Verywell Health,* November 2, 2019, https://www.verywellhealth.com>bedsore-in-a-nursing-home-3861403.

9 Quality of Care, 42 C.F.R. § 483.25, https://www.govregs.com/regulations/title42_chapterIV_part483_subpartB_section483.25.

10 Bursack, "About Bed Sores."

11 "Bedsores (pressure ulcers)," Patient Care & Health Info, Mayo Foundation for Medical Education and Research, February 9, 2020, https://www.mayoclinic.org/diseases-conditions/bed -sores/symptoms-causes/syc-20355893.

12 Bursack, "About Bed Sores."

13 John Hale, "How Long Should Iowans Wait for a Call Button
    Response?" *Des Moines Register,* August 18, 2016, 1:00
    p.m. CT, https://www.desmoinesregister.com/story/opinion/
    abetteriowa/2016/08/18/how-long-should- elderly-iowans-wait-call-
    button-response/88901332/.

14 Linda Esposito, "Living Well with a Feeding Tube," *U.S. News and
    World Report,* December 21, 2016.

15 Jose Vega MD, PhD, "When You Should Decide on Feeding Tubes for
    a Loved One," *Verywell Health,* November 20, 2019, https://www.
    verywellhealth.com/stroke-recovery-feeding-tube-placement-3145999.

16 ——, "When You Decide."

17 "Tube Feeding: What You Need to Know," M. D. Anderson Cancer
    Center, November 2009, https://www.mdanderson.org/transcripts/
    patient-education/tube-feeding.html.

18 "Living with a Feeding Tube," WebMD Medical Reference, WebMD,
    LLC., September 15, 2019, https://www.webmd.com/digestive-
    disorders/living-with-feeding-tube#1.

19 Barbara Peters Smith, "Should Nursing Home Residents be Forced
    to Take Showers?" *Sarasota Herald-Tribune,* March 20, 2013,
    12:01 a.m. EDT, https://www.heraldtribune.com/article/LK/20130320/
    News/605223025/SH.

20 "Guidance for Bathing Patients with Dementia: Bathing Without
    a Battle," The Commonwealth Fund, January 2006, https://www.
    commonwealthfund.org/publications/newsletter-article/guidance-
    bathing-patients-dementia-bathing-without-battle.

21 "ADL Care, Grooming and Personal Hygiene," Quality of Care, Regents
    of the University of Minnesota, November 22, 2011, http://www.
    hpm.umn.edu/nhregsplus/NH%20Regs%20by%20Topic/Topic%20
    Quality%20of%2 0Care.html#top.

22 Tom Underwood, "Forgotten Seniors Need Time, Care," *Atlanta
    Journal-Constitution,* October 5, 2010.

23 Michael Schroeder, "How to Monitor the Care of a Loved One in a
    Nursing Home," *U.S. News and World Report,* June 20, 2017.

24 Lisa Esposito, "The Visitors' Guide to Nursing Homes," *U.S. News and
    World Report,* October 4, 2019.

25 Lisa Packer, "Nursing Homes and Hearing Aids: What You Need to
    Know," *Healthy Hearing,* March 27, 2018, https://www.healthyhearing.
    com/report/52521-Nursing-homes-and-hearing-aids-what-you-
    need-to-know.

26 Hill, "Nursing Home Optometry."

27 Elaine Howley, "Eye Exams in Nursing Homes," *U.S. News and World
    Report,* September 13, 2019.

28 "Theft and Loss" (PDF), National Consumer Voice for Quality Long-Term Care, https://theconsumervoice.org/uploads/files/long-term-care-recipient/THEFT-AND-LOSS-FACT- SHEET.pdf.

29 Packer, "Hearing Aids."

30 ——, "Hearing Aids."

31 "20 Stats to Know About Hospice Care in the US," News, WesleyLife, July 24, 2014, https://www.wesleylife.org/blog/news/20-stats-to-know-about-hospice-care-in-the-us.aspx.

32 "Hospice Care," Caregiving, Aging in Place, November 2019, https://aginginplace.org/hospice-care/.

33 WesleyLife, "20 Stats to Know."

34 Nidhi Gulati and Laura Ross Cordaro, "Overcoming Oral Hygiene Challenges in the Nursing Home," *Caring for the Ages* 18, no. 8 (August 2017): 3, https://doi.org/10.1016/j.carage.2017.07.004.

35 Frank Scannapieco, "Poor Toothbrushing is Putting Nursing Home Residents at Risk," *Undark*, October 1, 2019.

36 Pamela Van Arsdall and Joanna Aalboe, "Improving the Oral Health of Long-Term Care Facility Residents," *Decisions in Dentistry Journal*, (May 2016): https://decisionsindentistry.com/article/improving-oral-health-long-term-care-facility-residents/.

37 Scannapieco, "Poor Toothbrushing."

38 Arsdall and Aalboe, "Improving."

39 Barbara Smith and Michael Helgeson, "Paying for Dental Work in Long Term Care," *Provider*, March 2013, 44.

40 Bridget Malkin, "Nail Cutting is an Essential Part of Nursing," *Nursing Times,* July 15, 2008.

41 Scannapieco, "Poor Toothbrushing."

42 Sarah Blanchard, "6 Signs of Nursing Home Neglect: Watch for These Red flags to Keep Your Loved One Safe and Healthy," Health, Next Avenue, February 18, 2016, https://www.nextavenue.org/6-signs-of-nursing-home-neglect/.

43 Mollie Durkin, "An Order Not to Hospitalize," *ACP Hospitalist,* https://acphospitalist.org/archives/2017/08/q-and-a-do-not-hospitalize.htm.

44 "Understanding the Difference Between DNR and DNH Advance Directives," Adult Care Advisors, May 5, 2014, https://www.adultcareadvisors.com/understanding-the-difference-between-dnr-and-dnh-advance-directives/.

45 Michael Schroeder, "A Lesser Known Advanced Directive: Do Not Hospitalize," *U.S. News and World Report,* June 8, 2017.

46 Resident Rights, 42 C.F.R. § 483.10(g)(2)(i)(ii), https://www.govregs.com/regulations/title42_chapterIV_part483_subpartB_section483.10.

47 S. F. Simmons, E. N. Peterson, and C. You, "The Accuracy of Monthly Weight Assessments in Nursing Homes: Implications for the Identification of Weight Loss," *Journal of Nutritional Health Aging* 13, no. 3 (March 2009): 284–288, https://doi.org/ 10.1007/s12603-009-0074-1.

48 Ann Brenoff, "Want Control Over Your Death? Consider a 'Do Not Hospitalize' Order," *The Huffington Post,* July 14, 2017, 8:31 a.m. EDT, https://www.huffpost.com/entry/do-not-hospitalize-orders_n_59666c35e4b0a0c6f1e54ed9.

49 ———, "Want Control."

50 Lori Johnston, "How to Know if a Parent is Eating in the Senior Living Community," AgingCare, https://www.agingcare.com/articles/determine-if-senior-in-senior-living-is-eating- 154464.htm.

51 "Nursing Homes: Improved Oversight Needed to Better Protect Residents from Abuse," U.S. Government of Accountability Office, June 13, 2019, https://www.gao.gov/products/GAO-19-433.

52 "Reporting Nursing Home Abuse: How to Report Abuse in Nursing Homes," Nursing Home Abuse Center, February 5, 2020, https://www.nursinghomeabusecenter.com/nursing-home-abuse/reporting-nursing-home-abuse/.

53 Bruce Y. Lee, "You May Lose Rights to Sue Nursing Homes, If Obama's Rule Is Overturned," *Forbes,* August 7, 2017.

54 "Nursing Home Abuse Statute of Limitations: Understanding the Statute of Limitations," Nursing Home Abuse Center, November 14, 2019, https://www.nursinghomeabusecenter.com/legal/statute-limitations/.

55 "New Rule Once Again Allows Nursing Home Arbitration Agreements," ElderLawNet, Inc., October 24, 2019, https://www.elderlawanswers.com/new-rule-once-again-allows-nursing-home-arbitration-agreements-17278.

56 "Medicare and Medicaid Programs; Revision of Requirements for Long-Term Care Facilities Arbitration Agreements (CMS-3342-F)," Centers for Medicare and Medicaid Services, July 16, 2019, https://www.cms.gov/newsroom/fact-sheets/medicare-and-medicaid-programs-revision-requirements-long-term-care-facilities-arbitration.

57 Jeffrey Pitman and Katherine Metzger, "Nursing Home Abuse and Neglect and the Nursing Home Reform Act: An Overview," *National Academy of Elder Law Attorneys Journal,* (October 2018): https://www.naela.org/NewsJournalOnline/OnlineJournalArticles/OnlineOct2018/NHAbuse.asp x.

58 ———, "Nursing Home Abuse."

59 "Signs of Nursing Home Abuse: Common Nursing Home Abuse Signs," Nursing Home Abuse Center, November 21, 2019, https://www.nursinghomeabusecenter.com/nursing-home- abuse/signs/.

60 Portia Wofford, "Nurses Say Staffing Ratios in Long Term Care
    Facilities Are Unsafe," Nurse.org, July 11, 2019, https://nurse.org/
    articles/nurse-staffing-unsafe-long-care-facilities/.
61 "Licensed Practical Nursing: Education Requirements, Career Paths
    & Job Outlook," All Nursing Schools, https://www.allnursingschools.
    com/licensed-practical-nurse/.
62 "Understaffing: Understaffing in the Nursing Home," Nursing
    Home Abuse Center, November 14, 2019, https://www.
    nursinghomeabusecenter.com/nursing-home-neglect/understaffing/.
63 Wofford, "Staffing Ratios."
64 "What Nursing Home Staff Levels Are Required?" ElderLawNet,
    Inc., May 23, 2017, https://www.elderlawanswers.com/what-nursing-
    home-staff-levels-are-required-6496.
65 Wofford, "Staffing Ratios."
66 ElderLawNet, Inc., "Staff Levels."
67 Alex Kacik, "Nursing Home Staffing Levels Often Fall Below CMS
    Expectations," *Modern Healthcare*, July 1, 2019.
68 Jordan Rau, "Like a Ghost Town: Erratic Nursing Home Staffing
    Reveled Through New Records," *Washington Post*, July 13, 2018,
    5:16 a.m. EDT, https://www.washingtonpost.com/national/health-
    science/like-a-ghost-town-erratic-nursing- home-staffing-revealed-
    through-new-records/2018/07/13/62513d62-867d-11e8-9e06-
    4db52ac42e05_story.html.
69 ——, "Ghost Town."
70 ——, "Ghost Town."
71 Alex Spanko, "75% of Nursing Homes 'almost never' in Compliance
    with RN Staffing Levels," *Skilled Nursing News*, July 1, 2019.
72 Rau, "Ghost Town."
73 ——, "Most Nursing Homes are not Adequately Staffed, New
    Federal Data Says," *PBS NewsHour*, July 13, 2018, 11:19 a.m. EDT,
    https://www.pbs.org/newshour/health/most-nursing- homes-are-not-
    adequately-staffed-new-federal-data-says.
74 Spanko, "75% of Nursing Homes."
75 Rau, "Ghost Town."
76 Marisa Kwiatkowski et al., "A national disgrace: 40,600 deaths tied
    to U.S. nursing homes," *USA Today*, June 2, 2020, 3:48 p.m. ET,
    https://www.usatoday.com/story/news/incestigations/2020/06/01/
    coronavirus-nursing-home- deaths-top-40-600/5273075002/.
77 Bryant Furlow, Carli Brosseau, and Isaac Arnsdorf, "Nursing Homes
    Fought Federal Emergency Plan Requirements for Years. Now, they're
    coronavirus hot spots," *ProPublica*, May 29, 2020.
78 Furlow, Brosseau, and Arnsdorf, "Nursing Homes Fought."
79 ——, "Nursing Homes Fought."
80 ——, "Nursing Homes Fought."

81 Rob Hayes and Grace Manthey, "Most CA nursing homes with COVID-19 cases were cited for infectious disease issues," ABC7 News online, April 22, 2020,-covid-19-inspections-infectious-disease-plan/6120040/.

82 Avik Roy, "The most important coronavirus statistic: 42% of U.S. deaths are from 0.6% of the population," *Forbes*, May 26, 2020.

83 Laura Strickler, "Trump admin won't require nursing homes to count Covid-19 deaths that occurred before May 6," NBC News, May 22, 2020, https://news.yahoo.com/trump-admin-wont-require-nursing-214349171.html.

84 Roy, "important coronavirus statistic."

85 Peter Whoriskey et al., "Hundreds of nursing homes ran short on staff, protective gear as more than 30,000 residents died during pandemic," *Washington Post*, June 4, 2020, https://washingtonpost.com/business/2020/06/04/nursing-homes-coronavirus-deaths/.

86 Ina Jaffe, "Ideal Nursing Homes: Individual rooms, better staff, more accountability," National Public Radio, May 21, 2020, https://www.npr.org/2020/05/21/855821083/ideal-nursing-homes-individual-rooms-better-staffing-more-accountability.

87 ——, "Ideal Nursing Homes."

88 Steven Reinberg, "Nursing Homes a Hotspot for Covid-19 Deaths," *U.S. News and World Report,* June 5, 2020.

89 "No sign of coronavirus? Here's why you could still be carrying (and spreading) it," Cleveland Clinic, May 6, 2020, https://health.clevelandclinic.org/studies-show-carriers-with-mild-or-no-symptons-are-key-part-of-covid-19-spread/.

90 Whoriskey et al., "short on staff."

91 Jaffe, "Ideal Nursing Homes."

92 Whoriskey et al., "short on staff."

93 Jaffe, "Ideal Nursing Homes."

94 Whoriskey et al., "short on staff."

95 ——, "short on staff."

96 Tony Pugh, "Abuse and Neglect at Nursing Homes Spur Calls for More Nurses," *Health Law & Business News,* August 15, 2019, 5:31 a.m. EDT, https://news.bloomberglaw.com/health-law-and-business/abuse-and-neglect-at-nursing-homes-spur-calls-for-more-nurses?context=search&index=2.

97 Wofford, "Staffing Ratios."

98 Nursing Services, 42 C.F.R. § 483.35(a), https://www.govregs.com/regulations/title42_chapterIV_part483_subpartB_section483.35.

99 Wofford, "Staffing Ratios."

100 Charlene Harrington, "The Need for Higher Minimum Staffing Standards in U.S. Nursing Homes," *Health Service Insights* 9, (April 2016): 13–19, https://doi.org/10.4137/HSI.S38994.

101 Wofford, "Staffing Ratios."

102 David Hefner, "Understaffed Nursing Homes Affecting Patients," *Journal of the National Medical Association* 94, no. 5 (May 2002): 283, https://www.ncbi.nlm.nih.gov/pmc/articles/PMC2594332/.

103 "Elder Abuse," Newsroom, World Health Organization, June 15, 2020, https://www.who.int/news-room/fact-sheets/detail/elder-abuse.

104 Lateshia Beachum, "Elderly care staff accused of running a dementia fight club, pitting patients against each other," *Washington Post,* October 16, 2019, https://www.washingtonpost.com/health/2019/10/14/elderly-care-staff-accused-pitting-residents-against-each-other-dementia-fight-club/.

105 Harrington, "Higher Minimum Staffing."

106 Jack Shea, "Man whose mother was abused by aides pushes for state lay to allow cameras in all nursing homes," FOX8 News, January 14, 2020, https://fox8.com/news/man-whose-mother- was-abused-by-aides-pushes-for-state-law-to-allow-cameras-in-all-nursing-homes/.

107 Philip Caulfield, "Man plants camera in elderly mother's nursing home, captures brutal abuse by caregivers," *New York Daily News,* June 29, 2011, 1:04 p.m. EDT, https://www.nydailynews.com/news/national/man-plants-camera-elderly-mother-nursing-home-captures-brutal-abuse-caregivers-video-article-1.125509.

108 "Nursing home cameras: more harm than good?" *Nursing Home Abuse Center Blog,* October 23, 2019, https://www.nursinghomecenter.com/blog/cameras-in-nursing-homes/.

109 David Grabowski "Mental Illness in Nursing Homes: Variations Across States," *Health Affairs* 28, no. 3 (May 2009): 689–700, https://doi.org/10.1377/hlthaff.28.3.689.

110 Wofford, "Staffing Ratios."

111 "NJ A382 Establishes Minimum Certified Nurse Aide-to-Resident Ratios in Nursing Homes," Bill Track 50, December 12, 2019, https://www.billtrack50.com/BillDetail/921999.

112 "CNA Salary in the United States," Salary.com, https://www.salary.com/research/salary/alternate/cna-salary.

113 Lois A. Bowers, "Assisted Living Will Need to Fill 1.2 Million Direct Care Jobs Over Next Decade," *Senior Living,* January 22, 2020, https://www.mcknightsseniorliving.com/home/news/assisted-living-will-need-to-fill-1-2-million-direct-care-jobs-over-next-decade-report/.

114 Charlene Harrington, "Does Investor Ownership of Nursing Homes Compromise the Quality of Care?" *American Journal of Public Health* 91, no. 9 (September 2001): 1452–1455, https://doi.org/10.2105/ajph.91.9.1452.

115 ——, "Higher Minimum Staffing."
116 "Non-Profit vs. For-Profit Nursing Homes: Is there a Difference in Care?" Article, Center for Medicare Advocacy, March 15, 2012, https://medicareadvocacy.org/non-profit-vs-for-profit- nursing-homes-is-there-a-difference-in-care/.
117 Allison Inserro, "For-Profit Nursing Home Residents Show More Signs of Neglect, Study Says," *American Journal of Managed Care*, (October 2018), https://www.ajmc.com/view/forprofit-nursing-home-residents-show-more-signs-of-neglect- study-says.
118 "Nursing Homes and Long-Term Care Facilities Industry Profile," Dun & Bradstreet First Research, May 27, 2020, http://www.firstresearch.com/Industry-Research/Nursing-Homes-and-Long-Term-Care-Facilities.html.
119 General Provisions, 42 C.F.R. § 488.402-456, https://www.govregs.com/regulations/title42_chapterIV_part488_subpartF_section488.402.
120 David Stevenson, "The Future of Nursing Home Regulation: Time for a Conversation?" *Health Affairs,* https://doi.org/10.1377/hblog20180820.660365.
121 Harrington, "Higher Minimum Staffing."
122 Stevenson, "Nursing Home Regulation."
123 Harrington, "Higher Minimum Staffing."
124 Harrington, "Higher Minimum Staffing."
125 "Association Releases 2019 State of the Restaurant Industry Report," National Restaurant Association, April 8, 2019, https://www.restaurant.org/articles/news/association-report-analyzes-industry-trends.
126 Carolyn Rosenblatt, "Outrageous! Nursing Home Illegally Dumps Elderly Resident They Don't Want," *Forbes,* November 2, 2017.
127 "Involuntary Transfer and Discharge in Nursing Homes," U.S. Department of Health and Human Services: Office of the Inspector General, https://oig.hhs.gov/reports-and-publications/workplan/summary/wp-summary-0000331.asp.
128 Jocelyn Wiener, "When Nursing Homes Push Out the Poor and Disabled Patients," *Washington Post*, December 20, 2017, https://www.washingtonpost.com/national/health-science/when-nursing-homes-push-out-poor-and-disabled-patients/2017/12/20/af9165ee-e56e- 11e7-927a-e72eac1e73b6_story.html.
129 Admission, Transfer, and Discharge Rights, 42 C.F.R. § 483.15(c)(1)(i), https://www.govregs.com/regulations/title42_chapterIV_part483_subpartB_section483.15.
130 K. Gabriel Heiser, "Nursing Home Discharges: Residents Have Rights," AgingCare, https://www.agingcare.com/articles/patient-rights-and-nursing-home-discharges-205724.htm.

131 Provision of a Hearing and Appeal System, 42 C.F.R. § 483.204, https://www.govregs.com/regulations/title42_chapterIV_part483_subpartE_section483.204.

132 Heiser, "Nursing Home Discharges."

133 Katie Engelhart, "Some Nursing Homes are Illegally Evicting Elderly and Disabled Residents Who Can't Afford to Pay," NBC News, November 29, 2019, 4:30 a.m. EST, https://www.nbcnews.com/news/us-news/some-nursing-homes-are-illegally-evicting-elderly-disabled-residents-who-n1087341.

134 Methods of Administration, 42 C.F.R. § 431.15, https://www.govregs.com/regulations/title42_chapterIV_part431_subpartA_section431.15.

135 Engelhart, "Illegally Evicting."

136 ——, "Illegally Evicting."

137 Wiener, "Push Out the Poor."

138 Engelhart, "Illegally Evicting."

139 ——, "Illegally Evicting."

140 Grabowski, "Mental Illness."

141 ——, "Mental Illness."

142 Engelhart, "Illegally Evicting."

143 Wiener, "Push Out the Poor."

144 Tara Siegel Bernard and Robert Pear, "How to Challenge a Nursing Home Eviction Notice," *New York Times*, February 22, 2018, https://www.nytimes.com/2018/02/22/business/nursing-home-eviction-rights.html.